ARTHRITIC COOKBOOK

HAMLYN DIETPLAN SERIES

Arthritic Cookbook

*

MARY LAVER

MARGARET SMITH

HAMLYN

The following titles are also available in this series:

Cooking for a Healthy Baby · Diabetic Cookbook
Low-fat Cookbook · Low-sodium Cookbook

The following titles are available in the Hamlyn Cookshelf series:

Biscuits and Cookies · The Chilli Cookbook
Cooking with Yogurt · Food Processor Cookbook
Mighty Mince Cookbook · Potato Cookery · Sweets and Candies

This book is dedicated to you the reader

The publishers would like to thank the following for lending the
tableware shown in the photographs:
Perrings   Reject Shop
Dickens and Jones, Richmond and other branches

Front cover photography by Longham Wood
Inside photography by David Johnson
Illustrations by Sue Lines

First published in 1981 by Pan Books Ltd.
This edition published in 1983 by
Hamlyn Publishing
a division of The Hamlyn Publishing Group Limited
Bridge House, London Road, Twickenham, Middlesex, England
© Copyright text Mary Laver and Margaret Smith 1981
© Copyright line illustrations and colour photographs
The Hamlyn Publishing Group Limited 1983

Fourth impression 1985

ISBN 0 600 32338 2

Set in Monophoto Bembo
by Photocomp Limited, Birmingham, England

Printed in Yugoslavia

CONTENTS

USEFUL FACTS AND FIGURES

Notes on metrication

In this book quantities are given in metric and Imperial measures. Exact conversion from Imperial to metric measures does not usually give very convenient working quantities and so the metric measures have been rounded off into units of 25 grams. The table below shows the recommended equivalents.

Ounces	Approx. g to nearest whole figure	Recommended conversion to nearest unit of 25	Ounces	Approx. g to nearest whole figure	Recommended conversion to nearest unit of 25
1	28	25	11	312	300
2	57	50	12	340	350
3	85	75	13	368	375 `
4	113	100	14	396	400
5	142	150	15	425	425
6	170	175	16 (1 lb)	454	450
7	198	200	17	482	475
8	227	225	18	510	500
9	225	250	19	539	550
10	283	275	20 ($1\frac{1}{4}$ lb)	567	575

Note: When converting quantities over 20 oz first add the appropriate figures in the centre column, then adjust to the nearest unit of 25. As a general guide, 1 kg (1000 g) equals 2.2 lb or about 2 lb 3 oz. This method of conversion gives good results in nearly all cases, although in certain pastry and cake recipes a more accurate conversion is necessary to produce a balanced recipe.

Liquid measures The millilitre has been used in this book and the following table gives a few examples.

Imperial	Approx. to nearest whole figure	Recommended ml	Imperial	Approx. ml to nearest whole figure	Recommended ml
$\frac{1}{4}$ pint	142	150 ml	1 pint	567	600 ml
$\frac{1}{2}$ pint	283	300 ml	$1\frac{1}{2}$ pints	851	900 ml
$\frac{3}{4}$ pint	425	450 ml	$1\frac{3}{4}$ pints	992	1000 ml (1 litre)

Spoon measures All spoon measures given in this book are level unless otherwise stated.

Can sizes At present, cans are marked with the exact (usually to the nearest whole number) metric equivalent of the Imperial weight of the contents, so we have followed this practice when giving can sizes.

Oven temperatures

The table below gives recommended equivalents.

	°C	°F	Gas Mark		°C	°F	Gas Mark
Very cool	110	225	$\frac{1}{4}$	Moderately hot	190	375	5
	120	250	$\frac{1}{2}$		200	400	6
Cool	140	275	1	Hot	220	425	7
	150	300	2		230	450	8
Moderate	160	325	3	Very hot	240	475	9

Notes for American and Australian users

In America the 8-oz measuring cup is used. In Australia metric measures are now used in conjunction with the standard 250-ml measuring cup. The Imperial pint, used in Britain and Australia, is 20 fl oz, while the American pint is 16 fl oz. It is important to remember that the Australian tablespoon differs from both the British and American tablespoons; the table below gives a comparison. The British standard tablespoon, which has been used throughout this book, holds 17.7 ml, the American 14.2 ml, and the Australian 20 ml. A teaspoon holds approximately 5 ml in all three countries.

British	American	Australian
1 teaspoon	1 teaspoon	1 teaspoon
1 tablespoon	1 tablespoon	1 tablespoon
2 tablespoons	3 tablespoons	2 tablespoons
$3\frac{1}{2}$ tablespoons	4 tablespoons	3 tablespoons
4 tablespoons	5 tablespoons	$3\frac{1}{2}$ tablespoons

An Imperial/American guide to solid and liquid measures

	Imperial	American		Imperial	American
Solid	1 lb butter or		Liquid	$\frac{1}{4}$ pint liquid	$\frac{2}{3}$ cup liquid
	margarine	2 cups		$\frac{1}{2}$ pint	$1\frac{1}{4}$ cups
	1 lb flour	4 cups		$\frac{3}{4}$ pint	2 cups
	1 lb granulated			1 pint	$2\frac{1}{2}$ cups
	or caster sugar	2 cups		$1\frac{1}{2}$ pints	$3\frac{3}{4}$ cups
	1 lb icing sugar	3 cups		2 pints	5 cups ($2\frac{1}{2}$ pints)
	8 oz rice	1 cup			

Note: When making any of the recipes in this book, only follow one set of measures as they are not interchangeable.

INTRODUCTION

On 21st October 1974 at my local hospital my life took a drastic change with these words from the rheumatologist: 'I am afraid, Mrs Laver, it is bad news; you have rheumatoid arthritis.' The truth now had to be faced.

My problems had begun four months earlier when I had started to suffer slight stiffness and pain in my fingers. Tests and more tests were duly made upon me while my condition became progressively more painful. Finally, the numbing verdict was announced.

To me the worst aspect was the fear of the unknown that lay ahead. What help was there? What sort of life was I going to lead? How would I live with the pain and prospects of a lifetime of arthritis? I went home and took stock of my disability: I had pain, swelling and stiffness in my jaw, neck, parts of the spine, shoulders, wrists, hands, hips, knees, ankles and feet.

That evening I happened to be watching an interview on television with Jane Banks, the American co-author of a cookery book for arthritics. She spoke of how, as an arthritic, she had been recommended to an American doctor, Dr Colin H. Dong. He put her on a special diet which he had developed himself, which arrested her complaint and left her free from pain and stiffness.

It seemed a hard way out of my predicament, so I started off by searching for other ways of beating my complaint. I tried hot wax on my hands and feet, visiting an osteopath, wearing a copper bracelet, and experimenting with a variety of potions and lotions – in fact, I tried anything that had the slightest chance of working. I was clutching at straws. But my pains persisted, especially by night, which deprived me of rest and sleep.

One day, browsing through a bookshop, I happened to see Dr Dong's cookery book. I decided to investigate further. Christmas was approaching, so it seemed sensible just to bias my eating habits towards the diet until after the festivities. My New Year resolution was to adhere totally to the principles of the diet. I was inspired by one of Dr Dong's sayings: 'Eating is a habit; all you have to do is change the habit'. So true, but so difficult.

For the first two weeks on the diet there were no obvious signs of improvement but during the third week, while taking a bath, I noticed that the swelling in my knees had subsided. Gradually, the swelling in my hands and feet was reduced and I was able to walk without pain in my hips. As the pain eased, I cut down on my pain-killing tablets, and after five months I stopped taking them altogether.

Further tests were made which confirmed my improving condition. My biggest step was to go back to playing squash after only two months on the diet. In fact, life returned completely to normal, and the diet became second nature after about six months of experimentation and adaptation.

There have been many occasions when I have succumbed to the temptation to deviate from it in small ways. When one knows the resulting pain is only temporary such dietary diversions may well be worth the consequences. Only the individual can judge what is or is not worthwhile, and the ability to decide soon develops with experience.

Inevitably, the biggest impact the diet has had on my life has been in enabling me to indulge in the activities I enjoy – and even those I don't, such as housework! I really appreciate being able to walk, cycle and go sailing again, instead of just taking these pleasures for granted.

THE DIET

Before you try the diet consult your doctor: he knows you and your condition. If, for instance, you have another complaint besides rheumatoid arthritis or osteoarthritis, then a change in your present diet may not be a good idea. I am not connected in any way with the medical profession and it would be irresponsible of me to encourage you to try the diet without taking medical advice.

I am sure that at first you will question many aspects of the diet. You will read that you cannot eat meat nor take milk, and you will want to know what you can substitute for these foods. The whole principle behind this diet is the belief that we suffer an allergic reaction to some of the things we eat – fruit, for example, which is one of the foods most missed in the diet. This contains some energy-giving sugar, a small amount of protein and Vitamins A and C in varying amounts, depending on the variety of the fruit and its age. It also contains potassium, magnesium, iron and calcium in small amounts. All these things can be obtained from other foods in the diet.

To illustrate allergies of this kind, whenever I visit groups of people I always start off my talks by drinking a glass of milk, which makes my hands swell up in twenty minutes. This is a visual indication, proof before their eyes of a violent allergic reaction.

I am not trying to condemn meat, dairy products and fruit but I can assure you that for many arthritics like myself they are likely to induce pain and are best replaced by other equivalent sources of protein, vitamins and minerals. Anyone on a new diet is bound to question whether it is adequate, but essentially a balanced diet is one which contains sufficient quantities of nutrients (that is, protein, carbohydrate, fat, vitamins and minerals) to maintain body functions, repair body tissue and provide sufficient energy. There should be no need to take added vitamins if care is taken to serve daily portions of food from each of the following four groups:

1 Protein foods   These include fish, chicken, egg whites, pulses (peas, soya beans and lentils) and nuts. At least two portions of these foods should be served every day.

2 Vegetables   These contain some protein, carbohydrate, fibre and vitamins, depending on type and freshness. Two or three portions should be chosen every day, and these should include green vegetables.

3 Cereals or grains   Rice, oats and wheat, for example, are good sources of energy and contain a certain amount of protein and fibre. The amount you need in your daily diet will depend on appetite.

4 Fats   Margarine and vegetable oils contain vitamins A, D and E and have a high calorific value. They should be eaten in moderation every day. Unused fat is stored in the body – too much will lead to obesity.

The charts on pages 123–125 show the nutritional value of different foods which are allowed in this diet and will be a useful guide when you plan your meals.

Right at the beginning, you will have to decide whether you are prepared to give up your favourite foods in order to seek relief. In time, when you are feeling better, you can try adding different foods to find out if you get a reaction from them. Then you will know whether you can afford to relax from the diet occasionally. I sometimes do at parties, but not very much. I keep away from tomatoes, soup, alcoholic drinks (except beer and the occasional glass of wine). Diversions from the diet in the early stages can mean seventy-two painful hours. Make sure that you think it is worth it.

The diet will not cure arthritis but it should bring you relief from stiffness and pain. Everyone asks how long it will take for it to be effective. In my case it took two weeks; in your case it could be longer, but you should have a good idea in three to five weeks. When the diet is working, in most cases the sign will be a foul taste in the mouth. This is caused by the elimination of toxins from the system. The foul taste and accompanying mouth odour will clear as you get better and only reappear when you make the odd diversion. If at first the diet does not seem to be working, then look for the cause – it may be coffee, margarine, honey or even nuts.

Your daily menus need not be complicated, nor do they have to cost any more than they did before. Few people are prepared to go to great trouble to prepare each meal as though it were a feast and you can continue your style of cooking as before; all you need to do is to change some of the foods you cook, substituting some of the ingredients.

Buying processed food is out, but you do not have to be a superb cook to give yourself nourishing meals. Care should be taken always to read the labels, especially when choosing textured vegetable protein or ready-made nut mixtures. For instance, not all health food products are acceptable, as some contain chemicals such as monosodium glutamate.

If you read through the following pages of foods which *are* allowed, you will realise how varied the diet can be. Note the list of foods which may not be eaten and avoid them, substituting other ingredients where necessary.

If you have been on the diet for some time and still seem to be in pain, take a close look at the past few days and make sure you are not suffering from overwork or stress. Another cause, which sometimes produces headaches, could be the body reacting to the process of eliminating toxins, and of course deviations from your diet can also cause pain, especially in the early stages. A foul taste in the mouth is a good sign, however, as it shows that the system is clearing itself of the toxins. Pain should be greatly reduced or disappear completely as the foul taste passes off.

If in doubt, consult your doctor, DO NOT cut out medication without medical advice first.

Foods you can eat

Fish and seafood
All fish is a good source of protein, minerals and the B complex vitamins, and oily fish supply vitamins A, D and E. Those which are eaten whole, for example sprats, provide an excellent source of calcium. Fresh fish should have a fresh smell, rather like seaweed, bright eyes and a clearly marked body. Cook it as soon as possible after purchase because it does not store well.

Smoked fish is allowed, but those which are dyed to produce the colouring must be avoided. If the colour is running on the fishmonger's slab this is a sure sign that the fish has been dyed and not correctly smoked.

Canned fish may be eaten so long as it is packed in pure vegetable oil. Avoid all the varieties with tomato or some other sauce. Frozen fish retains all the nutritive value of fresh fish and is best cooked straight from the frozen state. Processed frozen fish products, however, such as fish fingers and fish coated in batter or breadcrumbs, contain anti-oxidants and other additives and these must be avoided. Fish has a freezer life of about two to three months, after which it loses much of its flavour.

Shell fish are also a good source of protein and add interest to the diet. The pickled varieties are not allowed. It is particularly important to buy shell fish really fresh and in season.

Chicken
When you are beginning to feel the benefit of the diet you can start to introduce chicken breast into your meals. It is best to begin by first introducing chicken stock. Commercial chicken soups and stocks in powder or cube form must be avoided as all these. preparations contain additives. It is not difficult to make your own stocks and soups and several of the recipes show you how.

Soya bean products
There are three types of soya products used in the recipes – soya flour, soya bean milk and textured vegetable protein, known as TVP. All soya products are high in protein and minerals. Vitamins A and B complex are also present, along with some fat and carbohydrate.

Soya flour is a yellowish flour which can be used to increase the protein value of other foods. Soya milk has the same properties as cow's milk but the taste is different. Soya milk can be made at home by whisking flour into water, or it can be bought ready mixed in cans and cartons. The concentrated milk should be diluted only when needed and in this way a tin will last for four to five days. Though soya milk can be added to tea and coffee the acidity of some coffees may cause it to curdle.

Textured vegetable protein (TVP), resembling either mince or chunks of meat, is manufactured from soya beans. It can be flavoured and used as a substitute for meat and, as such, adds greater variety to this diet. It is advisable to buy the unflavoured varieties as some of the flavoured ones contain monosodium glutamate and artificial flavourings. Spun soya protein is also available, shaped and moulded to look remarkably like steaks and pieces of chicken, and can be combined with vegetables and sauces in casseroles and stews.

Soya protein needs reconstituting before use. Vegetable or chicken stock, or even yeast extract, can be used at this stage as flavouring. Large pieces of TVP need soaking for two or three hours, small chunks for about half an hour to an hour, and mince for only a few minutes.

TVP products should not be included in the diet at the very beginning, but may be gradually introduced when a marked improvement in your physical condition is noticed.

Nuts
Nuts are an excellent source of protein, fat, minerals and fibre. Most nuts are acceptable and they can be used either whole or ground, but roasted and salted nuts packed in bags or tins contain monosodium glutamate and they can cause pain to arthritis sufferers.

The protein in nuts is assimilated by the body more easily when eaten with a certain amount of carbohydrate, such as bread or potatoes. Peanut butter is an excellent spread for bread, but remember to read the labels to make sure there are no unacceptable additives.

Sunflower seeds
These seeds have a rather unusual nutty flavour, but they are as nutritious as all other nuts.

Rice
Brown rice, the natural grain, contains carbohydrate, protein and minerals and most of the vitamin B complex. When rice is refined, the outer husk is stripped off and 80 per cent of the vitamin B content and a good proportion of the minerals are lost. The grain is then polished white. It makes sense to gain all the nutrient available by

buying and cooking the unpolished brown rice, which has an interesting nutty taste and more bite than white rice.

Vegetables

These will form the backbone of your diet. Vegetables are usually served as an accompaniment and not as a dish on their own, so to get the best from vegetable main dishes you may have to readjust a little.

A good source of vitamin C, most vegetables also contain small amounts of vitamins A and E, protein and minerals. As there is no fruit in this diet, vegetables must supply your daily requirement of vitamin C. This is one of the least stable vitamins and it can be destroyed very easily. Being water soluble, it is absorbed into the cooking liquid, so the longer the vegetables are cooked the more vitamin C is lost. A further loss can occur when vegetables are kept hot for more than a few minutes.

The answer is to buy and use vegetables which are as fresh as possible. Prepare them just before you want to cook them, and don't cut them up too small. Plunge them into boiling water, cook for the least amount of time and, if possible, use the cooking water for making gravy. Frozen vegetables have a good nutrient content but the vitamin C may be destroyed if they are allowed to defrost before cooking. Do not buy frozen vegetables in a ready-prepared sauce – this may contain ingredients not allowed on the diet.

Vegetable oils

A diet free from animal fat means that all the fat required for cooking must come from vegetable sources. It is best to use specific oils which are high in polyunsaturated fatty acids and this group includes the oils obtained from safflowers, sunflower seeds, soya beans and corn.

Most supermarkets produce their own blends of vegetable oils and solid vegetable fats, but they can sometimes contain some of the cheaper oils which are high in saturated fats and these are best avoided. Olive oil, which is high in saturated fats, is one which is best used in small quantities for its flavour, as in salad dressings and Mediterranean dishes.

All oils are rich in vitamin E and are a valuable source of energy.

Margarine

Margarine can be used within the diet, but the one you use must be chosen with care as the fats can be of animal or vegetable origin. Margarine is often flavoured with milk solids and the colouring can be artificial or natural. Choose a margarine made from 100 per cent pure vegetable oils free from milk solids (whey) and artificial colouring.

You may find that you are able to tolerate small amounts of luxury margarine but be prepared to reject margarine if you are not feeling as well as you would like. A substitute which is worth trying is a spread made by melting some white solid vegetable fat, adding to it a little corn oil and a few leaves of rosemary for flavouring. A little salt can be added if you like.

Egg whites

The pure albumen in egg whites is a simple protein which is perfectly acceptable within this diet, but the yolk contains a fair amount of animal fat and should not be eaten.

Many dishes can be made equally well without the egg yolk, but when it is essential a mixture of soya flour and pure vegetable oil can be substituted. This mixture has most of the properties of egg yolk and is a reasonable substitute for flavour.

Bread and flour

The best bread for you to eat is that which you make yourself. You can then be sure that the flour and other ingredients are suitable for your diet. Bread making does take time and effort, however, though with the aid of food mixer and a deep freeze you can make a large batch and freeze the rest for use later.

Wholemeal flour, made from 100 per cent of the grain, has a high bran content and although suitable for bread making, is rather heavy for making cakes and sponges. An 80 per cent extraction flour in which 20 per cent of the bran and wheat germ has been removed is lighter and more suitable for the purpose. Both are pure flours. Flour milled and sold with more than 20 per cent of its bulk removed contains additives to compensate for the loss. These include iron, vitamins, nicotinic acid and chalk which are acceptable for the arthritic diet, but other improvers and bleaches are often added and these must be avoided.

Buy your bread only from small independent bakers or health food shops where you can establish what flour has been used. The cut and wrapped standard white loaf contains certain additives which should be avoided by the arthritic.

Crispbreads

When you buy crispbreads, choose the variety carefully. It is important to read the labels as some are made with milk derivatives and some have chemical additives. But there are suitable ones on the market, often sold in health food or wholefood shops.

Salt

An important ingredient in cooking, salt enhances flavour and may also be used as a preservative. Iodised sea salt is best.

Herbs

All types of herb are acceptable, and they can be used to enliven many of the meatless dishes which would otherwise be rather plain. Many varieties can be grown from seed in your garden or in pots.

Sugar

Sugar is acceptable within this diet. Your body can assimilate it and it should not give you pain. Having said that, you should also note that an excess will not do you any good. Sugar is naturally widely available in many foods, so leaving sucrose out will not leave your diet deficient in energy. Both brown and white sugars contribute only energy value to the diet. Molasses contains a trace amount of vitamin B and small amounts of iron and calcium.

Honey

Honey is one and a half times sweeter than sugar, and it can add variety to the sweet side of your diet. However, some honeys may aggravate your complaint so if you do have an adverse reaction from a particular honey you will know to avoid it in future.

Wine in cooking

Although wine is too acidic for most arthritics, a little used in cooking is acceptable as the wine breaks down during the cooking processes.

Alcohol and soft drinks

A small glass of rye whisky is the drink which will give least problems but drink it with water or plain soda, as commercial mixers such as ginger ale can produce painful side effects.

Fruit juice is out – try carrot juice instead if you want a soft drink.

Tea and coffee

There are many different teas with a range of delicate flavours that are at their best when drunk without milk and these are particularly suitable for this diet. Decaffeinated coffee is perfectly acceptable.

Foods you may not eat

Meat in any form, including broth. The exception is chicken and chicken broth, which you may be able to eat occasionally (see page 13).

Fruit of any kind, including tomatoes

Dairy produce, including egg yolks (but whites are acceptable), milk, cheese, yogurt

Vinegar, or any other acid

Pepper

Chocolate and cocoa (for flavouring, carob powder may be substituted)

Dry roasted nuts (the process involves the use of monosodium glutamate)

Alcoholic beverages

Soft drinks

All additives, preservatives, chemicals, and especially monosodium glutamate. One exception to this rule is the lecithin in margarine.

Food additives

For the rheumatoid or osteoarthritic, chemical food additives can mean pain, so they must be avoided. Unfortunately, not everything is labelled. Fresh vegetables, for instance, may be sprayed or treated with chemicals. If at all practical, grow as many of your own vegetables as possible or buy those which have been organically grown.

It is important to read the labels on frozen chickens. These will tell you if the chicken has been injected with any chemicals. Try to buy as little mass-produced food as possible.

The most common groups of additives include preservatives, sulphur dioxide, antioxidants, emulsifiers and stabilisers, colourings, flavourings and solvents. Wines, beers, soft drinks and dried vegetables all contain sulphur dioxide. Antioxidants are used with oils and fats to prevent them turning rancid. Emulsifiers and stabilisers are used extensively in the food-processing industry to improve appearance and ensure that foodstuffs maintain their texture during transport and storage. Similarly colourings, used in the canning industry and in many processed foods, will appear on the label as permitted colourings, and should be avoided. Chemically used flavouring agents are also commonly used; two of the most widely used flavourings for processed TVP are monosodium glutamate and hydrolysed protein. These too should be avoided.

One other additive you may find listed on a packet label is a solvent. These solvents are used to carry the flavour right through the food and, like the flavourings, are best avoided.

Even though the quantities of these chemicals are very small, they can still cause pain for the arthritic. It is far better to use natural flavourings, such as a vanilla pod instead of vanilla essence and, of course, to avoid all ready-prepared foods. In avoiding these additives, a little longer spent in the kitchen is inevitable, I'm afraid, but the bonus will be the relief from pain.

Introduction to the recipes

Having read all about the diet, the time has now come to get started. It's a good idea to choose a date a week or so ahead, so that you will have time to choose your menus and get your shopping list worked out. If at all possible, get the rest of the family interested in the idea because you will need their support and understanding.

First, have a good look in your larder, sort out all the foods not allowed on the diet and place them on one side. Put all the foods you *can* eat together, so that they will not be muddled up with the forbidden things. To do this you will have to read all the labels on the tins, jars and packets.

Now read through the list of foods you can eat, and make a shopping list of the fish and vegetables you really like so that during the first week of the diet you can spoil yourself a little. The first week will be the worst, but as you begin to feel better you will be encouraged to continue.

As with any diet, it is important that the meals are as appealing as possible. The addition of herbs and spices, for example, play an important part in such a natural diet. Fresh herbs are, without doubt, the best ones to use and these can be grown in small pots in the house – for example, parsley, sage and thyme. Soy sauce is another useful flavouring ingredient, but remember to read the label to check for unwanted additives.

The recipes that follow cover soups and starters, main meals, suppers and snacks as well as baking. There are also menu ideas which will guide you in your choice of dishes and help you to plan a nutritious diet.

Soups and Starters

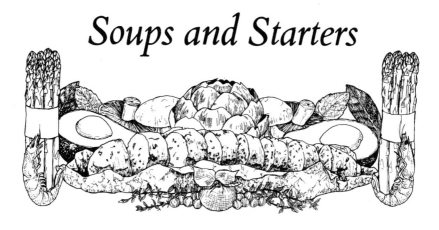

CHICKEN AND VEGETABLE SOUP

1 chicken breast joint	2 carrots, sliced
scant 1.15 litres/2 pints water	2 celery sticks, sliced
1 onion, finely chopped	1 small potato, diced
pinch of thyme	salt
2 parsley sprigs	pinch of nutmeg
1 bay leaf	chopped parsley to garnish

Place the chicken joint in a saucepan, cover with the water, then add the onion and the herbs. Bring to the boil, cover and simmer for an hour. Add the prepared vegetables to the pan and simmer for a further hour.

Remove the chicken joint from the stock. Cut all the meat off the bones, discard the skin and dice the flesh. Place the chicken meat in a clean saucepan. Strain the stock over the chicken.

Remove the bay leaf from the drained vegetables. Liquidise or press the vegetables through a sieve. For a coarse-textured soup, mash the vegetables with a potato masher. Add the resulting mixture to the stock and chicken in the saucepan. Reheat the soup, season with salt and a little nutmeg, and sprinkle with chopped parsley.

Serve very hot with Melba Toast or Croûtons (both on page 29). SERVES 4.

CHICKEN STOCK

1 onion, finely chopped
1 carrot, finely chopped
1 meaty chicken carcass or
    uncooked chicken joint

1.15 litres/2 pints water
bouquet garni

Place the vegetables in a saucepan with the chicken carcass or joint. Add the water and the bouquet garni and bring to the boil. Do not add salt when making stock as the long cooking time can give a salty result. Cover the pan, and allow to simmer for 1½ hours. Strain off the resulting stock and allow to cool.

This stock will keep in a refrigerator for up to 3 days, or it can be frozen and used as required.

Note: This stock can be used as a basis for making most of the soups in this book, but it is also useful for other dishes and as a flavouring for TVP.

It can be stored in a covered container in the refrigerator for up to 3 days or it may be frozen and used as required.

POTATO SOUP

450 g/1 lb potatoes, peeled and
    sliced
2 medium onions, chopped
2 large carrots, grated
1.75 litres/3 pints chicken stock
    (*above*)

1 teaspoon sugar
salt
pinch of nutmeg

Place the vegetables in a large saucepan, cover with the stock and season with sugar, salt and nutmeg. Bring to the boil, reduce the heat and cover the pan, then simmer for 1½ hours. Serve with thickly sliced wholemeal bread.

In spring and early summer, try adding about six finely chopped young nettle tops to the soup 10 minutes before it has finished cooking. Nettles combine well with potato. SERVES 4–6.

LEEK AND POTATO SOUP

4 leeks
25 g/1 oz margarine
450 g/1 lb potatoes, diced
25 g/1 oz plain flour

1.75 litres/3 pints chicken stock
    (page 21) or vegetable stock
salt
blade of mace

Trim the leeks, wash them well, and cut them into slices about 1 cm/ $\frac{1}{2}$ in thick. Melt the margarine in a saucepan and fry the leeks until lightly coloured; add the potatoes and cook for a further 5 minutes.

Stir in the flour and cook gently for 2 minutes, then remove from the heat. Gradually stir in the chicken stock and return the pan to the heat. Season with the salt and mace, then bring to the boil, cover the pan and simmer for 1 hour. Check the seasoning and remove the blade of mace before serving.

You can purée the soup in a liquidiser, adding a little extra stock to give it the required consistency. SERVES 4–6.

ONION SOUP

225 g/8 oz onions, finely sliced
40 g/1½ oz margarine
1 tablespoon plain flour

900 ml/1½ pints chicken stock
    (page 21)
2 bay leaves
salt

Fry the onions slowly in the margarine until golden brown and very soft. Stir in the flour and cook, stirring, for 5 minutes to brown the flour with the onions.

Remove from the heat, and gradually add the chicken stock. Bring to the boil, add the bay leaves and a little salt. Cover and simmer for 30 minutes.

Remove the bay leaves and serve the hot soup with crusty breads. SERVES 4.

CELERY SOUP

1 tablespoon oil
2 potatoes, diced
1 onion, diced
1 head of celery, trimmed,
   scrubbed and chopped

scant 1.15 litres/2 pints chicken
   stock *(page 21)* or water
1 bay leaf
½ teaspoon salt
chopped parsley to garnish

Pour the oil into a large saucepan, and fry the prepared vegetables in it for 2 minutes. Reduce the heat, cover the pan, and cook for 10 minutes to allow the flavours to mingle and make the vegetables soft, but not brown. Add the stock, bay leaf and salt; cover the pan and simmer for 1½ hours.

Strain the soup, reserving the liquid, and either liquidise the vegetables or pass them through a sieve. Return the vegetable purée to the soup liquid, reheat and season if necessary. Sprinkle a little chopped parsley over the soup before serving and offer a dish of Croûtons (page 29) as an accompaniment.

MUSHROOM SOUP

25 g/1 oz margarine
1 small onion, chopped
225 g/8 oz mushrooms, sliced
25 g/1 oz plain flour

300 ml/½ pint chicken stock
   (page 21)
450 ml/¾ pint soya milk
salt

Melt the margarine in a saucepan and add the onion. Cook until soft, but not brown. Add the mushrooms and cook for a further 2 minutes.

Stir in the flour and cook for another couple of minutes. Remove from the heat and gradually stir in the chicken stock and the soya milk. Return to the heat and bring to the boil, then cover and simmer for 30 minutes.

Add a little salt, if necessary, and serve hot with Melba Toast (page 29). SERVES 4.

ASPARAGUS SOUP

175 g/6 oz fresh asparagus
15 g/½ oz margarine
600 ml/1 pint chicken stock
  (page 21)

1 tablespoon cornflour
salt
soy sauce (optional)

Cut the asparagus into 5-mm/¼-in pieces and fry them in the margarine. Pour over the chicken stock, bring to the boil and simmer for 30 minutes.

Pour the soup into a liquidiser and process for 30 seconds. Strain through a sieve into a pan and reheat. Blend the cornflour with a little cold water and add this to the soup, stirring all the time. Bring to the boil, add a little salt and a little soy sauce. Serve hot with Croûtons (page 29). SERVES 2–3.

CORN AND TUNA SOUP

(Illustrated on page 34)

1 (99-g/13½-oz) can tuna fish
1 medium onion, chopped
50 g/2 oz long-grain rice

900 ml/1½ pints chicken stock
  (page 21) or vegetable stock
50 g/2 oz sweet corn, cooked

Heat 2 tablespoons of the oil from the can of tuna in a saucepan and add the onion. Fry until soft, then stir in the rice. Cook for 5 minutes, stirring occasionally. Stir in the stock, bring to the boil, cover the pan, and simmer for 25–30 minutes.

Place the contents of the saucepan in a liquidiser and blend until smooth. Return this to the saucepan, add the sweet corn and the flaked tuna fish. Heat through, and simmer for 5 minutes. Serve with Croûtons (page 29). SERVES 4.

CORN AND LENTIL SOUP

1 medium onion, sliced
1 medium potato, sliced
100 g/4 oz lentils
1.15 litres/2 pints chicken stock
 (page 21)

1 (396-g/11½-oz) can sweet corn
salt to taste

Put the onion, potato and lentils into a saucepan and pour in the stock. Bring to the boil and simmer for 30 minutes until the lentils are soft.

Strain off the stock into a clean pan, and transfer the lentils, potato and onion to a liquidiser. Add the sweet corn and process the mixture until smooth.

Return this purée to the pan containing the stock and reheat. Season with a little salt to taste and serve hot, garnished with chopped parsley. Croûtons (page 29) go very well with this soup to make it a substantial lunch dish. SERVES 4.

CUCUMBER AND PRAWN STARTER

1 teaspoon salt
½ cucumber, peeled and diced
1 small onion, finely grated
pinch of sugar

2 teaspoons chopped mint
2 tablespoons olive oil
225 g/8 oz peeled prawns
1 small lettuce, shredded

Sprinkle the salt over the cucumber and leave to stand for 30 minutes. Drain the liquid from the cucumber and add it, with the onion, sugar and the chopped mint, to the olive oil. Whisk the mixture to combine the ingredients.

Mix together the prawns and cucumber and place them on a bed of shredded lettuce on individual plates. Spoon over the dressing and serve well chilled with Walnut Bread (page 28). SERVES 4.

AVOCADO AND CRAB STARTER

2 ripe avocado pears
1 (198-g/7-oz) can crabmeat
angostura bitters

salt
pinch of paprika
watercress to garnish

Cut the avocado pears in half lengthways using a stainless steel knife so that the flesh will not be discoloured. Discard the stone in the middle and cut out the flesh. Do this as carefully as possible so that the skins are left in one piece. Neatly dice the flesh.

Mix together the drained crabmeat and the diced avocado pear, then season very lightly with angostura bitters and a little salt.

Pile the mixture back into the skins, sprinkle with a little paprika, and garnish with watercress. Serve with thin slices of brown bread and margarine. SERVES 4.

Note: It is important for their flavour that avocado pears are ripe when eaten. To test if an avocado is ripe, press the skin gently with your thumb; if the flesh feels hard the pear is not ripe but if the avocado feels slightly soft it is ripe. An avocado pear which feels very soft is either bruised or over-ripe. Hard avocados should be left in a warm place for 2–3 days to ripen.

MARINATED MUSHROOMS

225 g/8 oz button mushrooms
salt
1 clove garlic
4 tablespoons dry white wine
2 tablespoons olive oil

pinch of dried thyme or
  tarragon
2 parsley sprigs
1 bay leaf
12 coriander seeds

Wash the mushrooms and place them in a saucepan. Cover with water and add a little salt. Bring to the boil and simmer gently for 10 minutes. Drain the mushrooms and place them in a shallow dish.

Crush the clove of garlic and place it in a small saucepan. Add the rest of the ingredients. Bring to the boil and simmer for 10 minutes. Strain this mixture over the mushrooms, cover the dish and leave them to marinate for 24 hours.

When ready to serve, place the mushrooms in individual dishes and pour over a little of the strained marinade. Serve with crusty bread. SERVES 4.

MARINATED LEEKS

3 tablespoons oil
1 celery stick, chopped
4 leeks, cut into 2.5-cm/1-in
   pieces

450 ml/¾ pint chicken stock
   (page 21)
bouquet garni
10 coriander seeds

Heat the oil in a saucepan, add the celery, and cook for 2–3 minutes. Add the leeks and sauté these for 2 minutes.

Pour in the stock, add the bouquet garni and the coriander seeds, then bring to the boil. Simmer for about 15 minutes until the leeks are tender but not broken.

Drain the leeks carefully and arrange them in a serving dish. Strain a little of the cooking liquid and pour this over the vegetables, then cover and chill well.

Serve with crusty wholemeal bread for a starter or light lunch. Serves 2–4.

ARTICHOKES WITH MUSHROOMS

4 large globe artichokes
salt
4 tablespoons olive oil
2 cloves garlic, crushed

100 g/4 oz mushrooms, sliced
pinch of dried thyme
1 small lettuce, shredded

Trim off and discard the stems from the artichokes, wash them in plenty of water, then add them to a saucepan of boiling salted water. Reduce the heat, cover and cook for 40–45 minutes, or until the leaves pull away easily. Drain the artichokes upside down and allow to go cold.

Heat one tablespoon of the olive oil in a small saucepan. Add the garlic and mushrooms and cook for 5 minutes. Allow to go cold, then add the thyme, a little salt and the rest of the olive oil.

Pull off and discard the outer leaves of the artichoke until you come to the base which is surrounded by fine hairs. Remove the hairs and place the artichoke bottoms on a bed of lettuce. Pour over the mushroom and oil dressing and serve well chilled. Serves 4.

WALNUT BREAD

4 slices day-old wholemeal
  bread
margarine for spreading

50 g/2 oz walnuts, finely
  chopped
salt

Spread the bread with margarine and remove the crusts. Sprinkle the walnuts over the slices, and season them very lightly with salt. Place the slices on a dampened sheet of greaseproof paper and carefully roll up the bread like a Swiss roll. Wrap the rolls in the damp paper for 20 minutes, so that they will not unroll when sliced.

Cut the rolls into 5-mm/¼-in slices and serve the pinwheels with Cucumber and Prawn Starter (page 25). SERVES 4.

Sunflower Pinwheels
You can, if you like, make these pinwheels with lightly toasted, chopped sunflower seeds instead of the walnuts. Use 50 g/2 oz sunflower seeds and toast them lightly under a hot grill, turning frequently to prevent the seeds from burning.

Cucumber Pinwheels
Thinly peel a quarter of a large cucumber. Coarsely grate the cucumber and squeeze out all the liquid. Spread the grated cucumber over the bread and margarine and season lightly. Roll up and slice as above.

HERB BREAD

1 long thin loaf white bread
  (*page 114*)
75 g/3 oz margarine

1 teaspoon dried mixed herbs *or*
  2 teaspoons chopped fresh
  herbs

Cut the loaf into slices down as far as the bottom crust to keep the slices attached at the base. Cream the margarine and mix in the herbs.

Spread the margarine mixture on the slices. Re-form the loaf and spread a little extra margarine on top. Wrap the loaf in some foil and bake in a moderately hot oven (190c, 375f, gas 5) for about 15 minutes. Serve immediately. SERVES 6–8.

Note: If you are preparing herb bread using fresh herbs, try to use those herbs which will complement the main dish. For example, use a mixture of parsley and lemon balm if the bread is to be served with fish; try using tarragon and parsley or thyme to accompany chicken and use basil, oregano or marjoram with vegetables.

MELBA TOAST

Cut wafer-like slices of stale white or brown bread. Remove the crusts and place the bread in a moderately hot oven (200c, 400F, gas 6) for 10 minutes until crisp, dry and curled.

Melba toast goes well with most soups; serve it hot or cold with margarine.

Note: Alternatively, you can make melba toast under the grill but you must take care not to burn the bread. Lightly toast medium-thick slices of bread on both sides, then cut off the crusts and slice each piece horizontally in half to give two thin pieces, toasted on one side. Toast the uncooked sides under the hot grill; the bread will curl as it cooks.

CROÛTONS

2 slices white or wholemeal bread

a little corn oil

Cut the slices of bread into 5-mm/$\frac{1}{4}$-in cubes. Heat the oil and fry the cubes of bread until brown and crisp on all sides. Drain on absorbent kitchen paper.

Garlic Croûtons
Add a crushed clove of garlic to the oil in the pan before adding the bread. Continue as above.

Herb Croûtons
Sprinkle 2 teaspoons chopped fresh herbs over the hot croûtons and toss well.

Curry Croûtons
Sprinkle 1-2 teaspoons curry powder into the hot oil and cook for a minute before adding the bread, then continue as above. Serve these croûtons to pep up simple fish or vegetable dishes.

Fish and Seafood

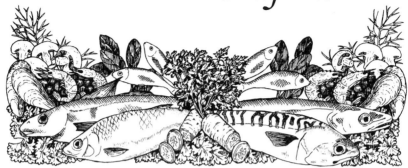

MUSSELS

2 kg/4½ lb fresh mussels
salt
450 ml/¾ pint water *or* 300 ml/
  ½ pint water and 150 ml/¼ pint
  dry white wine

1 onion, diced
1 small carrot, diced
2 parsley sprigs
1 tablespoon cornflour
chopped parsley to garnish

Mussels must be bought when really fresh and cooked on the same day.

Place the mussels in a large bowl and cover with cold water, add a little salt and leave until ready to cook. Carefully examine the mussels and throw away any with cracked or broken shells, or any which are open and do not shut immediately when tapped. Scrub the mussels with a stiff brush and remove the black 'beard' which is fixed to the side of the shell.

In a large saucepan mix the water or water and wine, the vegetables and the parsley. Bring this mixture to the boil and simmer for 10 minutes.

Place half the mussels in the pan, cover tightly, and allow to cook for 7–8 minutes, shaking the pan from time to time. At the end of this time remove them and cook the remainder of the mussels. At the end of 7–8 minutes cooking they will have opened and any that have not opened must be discarded.

Remove the mussels from their shells, place them in a soup tureen or large serving dish and cover with a cloth to stop them drying out. Keep hot until ready to serve.

Strain the cooking water through a muslin cloth into a clean saucepan. Mix the cornflour to a thin cream with a little water and add this to the saucepan. Bring to the boil, stirring all the time. Pour this over the mussels and sprinkle with parsley.

Serve immediately with crusty bread. SERVES 4.

CURRIED PRAWN RING

2 tablespoons olive oil
1 onion, chopped
450 g/1 lb long-grain rice
1 litre/1¾ pints chicken stock
  (page 21) or fish stock
25 g/1 oz margarine
1 teaspoon curry powder

25 g/1 oz plain flour
100 g/4 oz frozen peas
100 g/4 oz sweet corn
225 g/8 oz peeled prawns
salt
chopped parsley to garnish

Heat the oil in a saucepan, add the onion, and cook for 2–3 minutes. Stir in the rice and fry for 5 minutes. Carefully pour in 750 ml/ 1¼ pints of the stock, cover the pan and simmer the rice for 20 minutes until soft and all the liquid is absorbed. Grease a plain ring mould and firmly pack in the cooked rice. Keep warm.

Melt the margarine in a small saucepan, add the curry powder and cook for one minute, then add the flour and cook for two minutes more. Remove from the heat and gradually stir in the remaining stock. Return to the heat, bring to the boil, and cook until thick.

Cook the frozen peas and sweet corn in a little boiling salted water for five minutes. Drain and keep on one side. Add to the sauce with the cooked prawns. Simmer for five minutes and season with a little salt.

Carefully unmould the rice on to a serving dish, and spoon the prawn mixture into the centre of the ring. Sprinkle the top with a little parsley before serving.

Serve with a green or mixed salad. SERVES 6–8.

PRAWN SALAD

1 clove garlic
450 g/1 lb peeled prawns
1 celery stick, finely sliced
1 green pepper, finely sliced

1 lettuce
4 tablespoons Creamy Salad
 Dressing *(page 121)*

Cut the garlic in half and rub the cut side around the inside of a salad bowl to give a slight garlic flavour to the salad.

Remove any black veins from the backs of the prawns, and mix them with the celery and pepper. Arrange the washed, dry lettuce in the salad bowl and pile the prawn and vegetable mixture on top.

Just before serving the salad pour over the creamy salad dressing. Serve with some fresh wholemeal bread rolls. SERVES 6.

WHITEBAIT

225 g/8 oz whitebait
25 g/1 oz wholemeal flour
salt

parsley
oil for deep frying

Wash the whitebait in cold water and pat it dry on absorbent kitchen paper. Season the flour with a little salt and dip the fish in it, then shake off any excess.

Heat the oil to 180c/350f, plunge in the fish, a handful at a time, and cook for 2–4 minutes until they are crisp and golden brown. Drain on absorbent kitchen paper and keep hot whilst the rest of the fish are being cooked.

Tie some fresh parsley in a bunch with a piece of cotton and fry it in the hot oil until crisp.

Drain the parsley and use it to garnish the whitebait. SERVES 2–3.

Kedgeree (page 53) with Margo's Bread (page 114)
and Vegetable Cocktail (page 96)

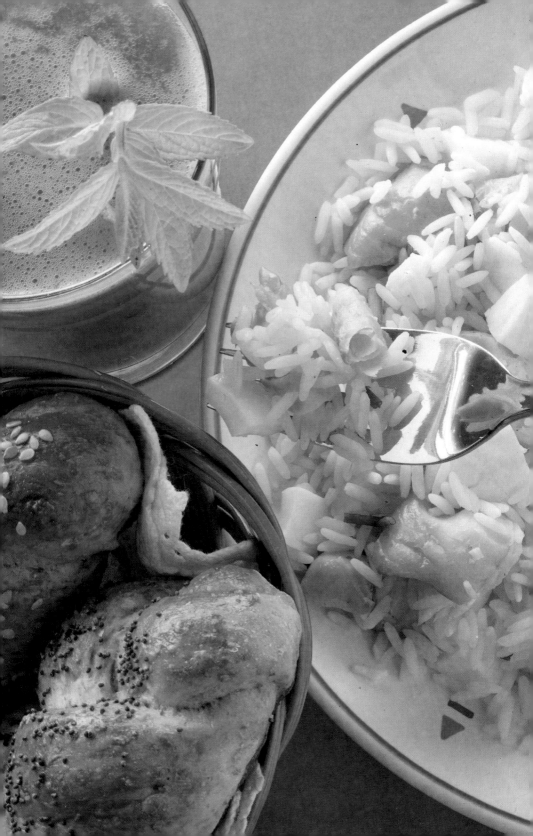

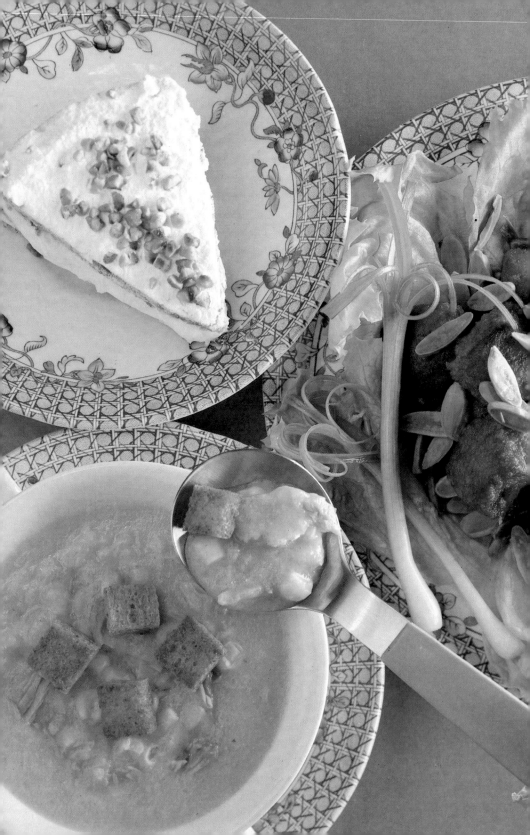

FRIED COD'S ROE

450 g/1 lb fresh cod's roe,
  washed
1 bay leaf
1 small onion, sliced
salt

100 g/4 oz fresh breadcrumbs
a little plain flour
1 egg white, lightly beaten
oil for shallow frying

It is possible to buy cod's roe ready boiled, but do make sure that it is really fresh as it dries out very quickly.

Place the roe in a saucepan and cover with cold water. Add the bay leaf and onion, plus a little salt. Bring slowly to the boil, cover the pan and simmer very gently for 15 minutes so that the roe does not break.

Take out the cooked roe and place in a small loaf tin or other container. Cover with greaseproof paper, place a weight on top and allow the roe to go cold. When cold and pressed, cut into thick slices.

Place the breadcrumbs on a flat plate, and place a little flour in a dish. Dip the slices of roe, first in the four, then in the egg white, and finally in the breadcrumbs. Press the coating on well.

Heat a little oil in a frying pan and fry the slices of roe until golden brown. Drain on absorbent kitchen paper. Serve with toast as a substantial snack for lunch or supper. SERVES 4.

Corn and Tuna Soup (page 24), Marinated Chicken with Almonds (page 63) and Hazelnut Meringue Cake (page 108)

PRINCE'S FISH PIE

15 g/½ oz margarine
4 anchovy fillets
450 g/1 lb cod fillet
EGG SAUCE
50 g/2 oz margarine
25 g/1 oz plain flour
150 ml/¼ pint each of white wine
  and water *or* 300 ml/½ pint
  soya milk

2 hard-boiled egg whites,
  chopped
POTATO TOPPING
675 g/1½ lb potatoes
25 g/1 oz margarine
nutmeg

Melt the 15 g/½ oz of margarine in a small pan, add the anchovies and cook, stirring, until the margarine and anchovies are well blended. Skin the fish fillets.

In another pan melt half the margarine for the sauce and stir in the flour. Cook, stirring, until the mixture bubbles. Remove from the heat and gradually add the wine and water or soya milk. Return to the heat and cook, stirring, until thickened. Beat in the remaining margarine, add the egg whites to the mixture and mix well.

Cook the potatoes in boiling salted water until tender, drain and mash them with the margarine and season with a little grated nutmeg. Grease a pie dish with margarine or oil and pour in half the egg sauce. Lay the cod fillet on top and spread the anchovy mixture over. Coat the remaining egg sauce.

Pipe or spoon the potato over the fish and bake in a moderate oven (180c, 350f, gas 4) for 45–50 minutes until the top is crisp and brown. SERVES 4.

TIPSY COD

450 g/1 lb cod fillet
50 g/2 oz mushrooms, sliced
40 g/1½ oz margarine
150 ml/¼ pint white wine

salt
25 g/1 oz plain flour
450 g/1 lb creamed potatoes
parsley sprigs to garnish

Cut the fish into 2.5-cm/1-in cubes and place them in a shallow ovenproof dish. Add the mushrooms, dot with about 15 g/½ oz of the margarine and pour over the white wine. Add a little salt. Cover the dish and bake in a moderately hot oven (190c, 375f, gas 5) for 25 minutes.

Melt the other 25 g/1 oz of margarine in a saucepan, add the flour and cook for two minutes. When the fish is cooked, strain off the liquid and add this to the flour and margarine. Bring to the boil and cook until thick. Add a little water if the sauce is too thick (it should be of a coating consistency). Pour the sauce over the fish. Cover with creamed potatoes and return to the oven for further 20 minutes to heat through and brown. Garnish with parsley before serving. SERVES 4.

BORDERED COD

450 g/1 lb cooked cod
25 g/1 oz margarine
3 anchovy fillets
25 g/1 oz plain flour
300 ml/½ pint soya milk or fish
   stock
1 tablespoon chopped parsley

100 g/4 oz peeled shrimps or
   prawn pieces
salt
450 g/1 lb potatoes
a little extra margarine
a little extra soya milk

Remove the skin and bone from the cod and flake the flesh.

Melt the margarine in a saucepan, add the anchovy fillets and cook, stirring until the fillets are broken up. Stir in the flour and cook for 2 minutes. Remove from the heat and gradually add the soya milk or fish stock, stirring all the time. Return to the heat and bring to the boil, then cook until thick. Add the chopped parsley, flaked fish, shrimps and salt to taste. Leave on one side.

Boil the potatoes in salted water until tender. Drain and mash. Beat in a little margarine and soya milk to make a soft potato mixture. Pipe or pile a border of the potato around a shallow heated serving dish.

Reheat the fish very carefully so that it does not break up and spoon the mixture into the centre of the serving dish. SERVES 4.

COD À LA MAÎTRE D'HÔTEL

450 g/1 lb cod
salt
blade of mace *or* 1 bay leaf

50 g/2 oz margarine
1 small onion, chopped
1 teaspoon chopped parsley

Place the cod in a saucepan, cover with cold water, and add a little salt plus the blade of mace or bay leaf. Cover the pan and bring slowly to the boil, then simmer very gently for 10 minutes, or until the fish flakes easily.

Melt the margarine in a large saucepan, add the onion and sauté for 3 minutes. Add the parsley.

Strain the fish and flake into large pieces, then add to the onion mixture. Very carefully toss the fish in the pan and reheat, taking care not to break it up too much.

Serve with mashed potatoes or rice. SERVES 4.

Note: Reserve the fish stock and use when needed in another recipe.

COD ITALIEN

25 g/1 oz margarine
1 clove garlic, crushed
1 tablespoon chopped chives
1 tablespoon chopped parsley
50 g/2 oz mushrooms, sliced
2 tablespoons plain flour

150 ml/$\frac{1}{4}$ pint white wine
3 tablespoons fish stock or water
salt
4 small cod fillets
oil for shallow frying

Melt the margarine in a saucepan, add the garlic, chives, parsley, and mushrooms. Cook for 3 minutes. Add 1 tablespoon of the flour and cook for 2 more minutes.

Mix together the wine and stock or water and gradually add this to the vegetable and herb mixture, stirring all the time. Season with salt, bring to the boil, and simmer for 10 minutes.

Add a little salt to the remaining flour and sprinkle it over the fish fillets. Heat some oil in a frying pan and fry the cod fillets until golden brown. Drain the fish on absorbent kitchen paper and place on a heated serving dish. Pour over the sauce and serve immediately. SERVES 4.

CURRIED COD

450 g/1 lb cod
salt
25 g/1 oz plain flour
50 g/2 oz margarine
1 onion, sliced

1 clove garlic, crushed
2 teaspoons curry powder
600 ml/1 pint fish stock or
   chicken stock *(page 21)*

Cut the cod into bite-sized cubes. Mix the salt with the flour and dip the cod pieces in this mixture.

Melt half the margarine in a frying pan and quickly fry the pieces of fish until golden brown. Place the fish in an ovenproof casserole.

Put the rest of the margarine in the pan, add the onion and garlic and cook until golden brown. Sprinkle in the curry powder and any flour left over from coating the fish, then cook for 2 minutes. Remove from the heat and stir in the stock, a little at a time. Return to the heat and bring to the boil.

Pour this sauce over the fish and place in a moderate oven (180c, 350f, gas 4) for 20 minutes to cook the fish through and to develop the curry flavour.

Serve with plain boiled rice. SERVES 3–4.

STUFFED COD STEAKS

25 g/1 oz margarine
1 large onion, finely chopped
100 g/4 oz mushrooms, finely
   chopped
2 tablespoons fresh breadcrumbs

$\frac{1}{2}$ teaspoon dried mixed herbs
salt
4 middle-cut cod steaks
2 tablespoons dry white wine or
   water

Melt the margarine in a saucepan, add the onion and sauté for 3 minutes until soft. Add the mushrooms and cook for a further 5 minutes. Remove the pan from the heat then add the breadcrumbs and herbs. Mix well and season with a little salt.

Remove the bones from the centre of the cod steaks and fill the cavities with the stuffing. Re-form the steaks and secure them with wooden cocktail sticks. Place in a greased ovenproof dish, and pour in the wine or water. Cover with foil and bake in a moderate oven (180c, 350f, gas 4) for 20–30 minutes or until the fish flakes easily. The time will depend on the thickness of the cod steaks. SERVES 4.

HERBY HADDOCK

4 haddock fillets
3 tablespoons oil
1 tablespoon white wine
$\frac{1}{2}$ teaspoon salt
1 tablespoon chopped fresh
    parsley

$\frac{1}{4}$ teaspoon dried thyme or a few
    fresh thyme sprigs
1 small onion, sliced
1 bay leaf

Place the haddock fillets in a shallow dish. Combine the oil and wine. Add the salt and herbs to make a marinade.

Sprinkle the onion over the fish and pour over the marinade. Add the bay leaf, cover the fish and leave in a refrigerator for at least 4 hours.

When ready to cook, drain the fillets from the marinade and place them under a preheated grill. Brush the fillets with the marinade during cooking to prevent them drying out. SERVES 4.

BASIL'S FILLETS

4 haddock fillets
2 tablespoons oil
salt
2 tablespoons chopped fresh
    parsley

$\frac{1}{2}$ teaspoon dried basil
a little plain flour
25 g/1 oz margarine
100 g/4 oz mushrooms, sliced

Place the fish fillets on a flat plate and brush them on both sides with half the oil. Sprinkle with a little salt and most of the chopped parsley. Lastly, sprinkle over the basil. Cover and leave in a cool place for at least half an hour (longer if possible) so that the fillets absorb the flavour of the herbs. When ready to cook, dredge the fillets with flour until evenly coated, leaving the herbs on the fish.

Melt the margarine and remaining oil in a frying pan and fry the fillets until golden brown on both sides, but do not overcook them. Keep hot. If necessary, add a little more margarine to the pan and slide in the mushrooms. Sprinkle over the remaining parsley, stir, then cover the pan and allow the mushrooms to cook in their own juices for 5 minutes.

Place a spoonful of the mushroom mixture on each fish fillet and serve with boiled or mashed potatoes and a green vegetable. SERVES 4.

BAKED HAKE IN OATMEAL

4 thick hake cutlets
2 onions, sliced
salt
50 g/2 oz fine oatmeal
25 g/1 oz margarine
1 tablespoon oil
1 large parsnip, diced
COURT-BOUILLON
1 onion, chopped

1 carrot, chopped
trimmings from the fish cutlets
    (skin and bone)
1.15 litres/2 pints water
1 thyme sprig
1 parsley sprig
1 bay leaf

First make the court-bouillon: add the onion and carrot, with the fish trimmings, to the water. Add the herbs and bring slowly to the boil. Cover and simmer for 30 minutes.

Rub the fish with a piece of cut onion and sprinkle with salt. Coat the fish in the oatmeal. Melt the margarine and oil in a frying pan and fry the fish until golden brown, but not cooked through. Remove the fish from the pan and place in an ovenproof casserole.

Fry the onion and parsnip in the remaining fat until golden brown. Add the vegetables to the fish in the casserole and pour over the strained court-bouillon. Cover and bake in a moderate oven (180c, 350f, gas 4) for 40 minutes. SERVES 4.

BAKED HAKE STEAKS

4 (175-g/6-oz) hake steaks
2 tablespoons plain flour
salt

1 small onion, finely chopped
1 teaspoon chopped parsley
1 tablespoon oil

Place the steaks in a greased ovenproof dish. Dredge them with the flour, season with salt and sprinkle over the onion and parsley. Sprinkle over the oil and cover the dish with a lid or foil.

Bake in a moderate oven (180c, 350f, gas 4) for 20 minutes. Remove the foil and increase the heat to moderately hot (200c, 400f, gas 6) for a further 10 minutes to brown the steaks.

Transfer the hake to a heated serving dish and strain over the liquid. Serve immediately. SERVES 4.

FOILED FISH

450 g/1 lb white fish fillets
25 g/1 oz margarine *or*
   1 tablespoon oil
salt

100 g/4 oz mushrooms, sliced
2 teaspoons chopped lemon
   balm or parsley

Cut pieces of foil, each one twice the size of each fish fillet, and brush with a little oil or grease with margarine.

Lay a fillet of fish on each piece of foil, sprinkle with a little salt, and cover with the mushrooms. Sprinkle over the lemon balm or parsley and pour on just a little oil or dot with margarine. Parcel up the foil to make neat little packages and seal the edges firmly, so that none of the natural juices are lost. Bake in a moderately hot oven (190c, 375f, gas 5) for 20–30 minutes.

It is best to serve the parcels unopened, so that they get to the table really hot with all the juices still in the package.

SAUCY FISH

50 g/2 oz margarine
50 g/2 oz plain flour
600 ml/1 pint soya milk
salt
2 tablespoons chopped parsley

450 g/1 lb white fish fillets
100 g/4 oz mushrooms
450 g/1 lb potatoes, thickly sliced
a little margarine or oil

Melt the margarine in a saucepan, sprinkle in the flour, and cook for 2 minutes. Remove from the heat and stir in the soya milk a little at a time to make a smooth sauce. Return to the heat and cook until thickened. Season with a little salt and add the chopped parsley.

Pour half this sauce into a greased 2-litre/3½-pint casserole and lay the fillets of fish on top. Sprinkle over the sliced mushrooms and then pour in the rest of the sauce.

Place the potato slices in cold salted water. Cover and bring to the boil, then reduce the heat and simmer for 15 minutes. Drain the potatoes and arrange them over the top of the casserole. Sprinkle over a little oil, or dot with margarine, and bake in a moderately hot oven (190c, 350f, gas 5) for 45–50 minutes. SERVES 4.

BAKED FISH WITH MUSHROOMS

50 g/2 oz margarine
1 tablespoon chopped parsley
salt

450 g/1 lb white fish fillets
225 g/8 oz mushrooms, sliced
2–3 tablespoons white wine

Cream the margarine, mix in the parsley and season with a little salt. Place the fish fillets in a greased baking dish and cover with the sliced mushrooms. Sprinkle over the wine and dot with parsley margarine.

Cover and bake in a moderate oven (180c, 350f, gas 4) for 20 minutes. SERVES 4.

FISH SHELLS

double quantity Short Crust
 Pastry *(page 112)*
25 g/1 oz margarine
25 g/1 oz plain flour
300 ml/½ pint soya milk or fish
 stock

225 g/8 oz white fish, cut into
 small cubes
salt
a little powdered mace
1 tablespoon chopped parsley

Grease six scallop shells. Roll out half the pastry thinly and use this to line the shells. Press in the pastry firmly so that the impressions of the shells are made in the pastry.

Melt the margarine in a saucepan. Add the flour and cook for 2 minutes. Remove from the heat and gradually add the soya milk or fish stock, stirring all the time. Return to the heat, bring to the boil, and cook until thick. Add the fish cubes to the sauce with the salt, powdered mace and the chopped parsley. Allow the mixture to cool. Divide the mixture between the six lined shells. Roll out the other half of the pastry and cover the shells with pastry lids. Dampen the edges to make sure the lids are firmly attached.

Bake in a moderately hot oven (200c, 400f, gas 6) for 20 minutes or until the pastry has set. Carefully unmould the pastry from the shells; turn upside down so that the shell markings are uppermost and return to the oven for a further 15 minutes until the pastry is golden brown. Serve hot or cold. SERVES 6.

CASSEROLE OF FISH

450 g/1 lb white fish
1 tablespoon plain flour
generous pinch of paprika
salt
1 small red pepper, finely sliced
1 small green pepper, finely
    sliced

1 onion, sliced
100 g/4 oz sweet corn
1 bay leaf
300 ml/½ pint fish stock

Cut the fish into bite-sized pieces. Mix together the flour, paprika and salt. Coat the fish in this mixture.

Layer the fish, peppers, onion and sweet corn in an ovenproof casserole, add the bay leaf and pour over the fish stock. Cover and bake in a moderate oven (180c, 350f, gas 4) for 45 minutes.

Serve with potatoes and a green vegetable. SERVES 4.

WHITE FISH AND CORN PIE

(Illustrated on page 51)

450 g/1 lb white fish
salt
bouquet garni
2 tablespoons oil
1 clove garlic, crushed
1 onion, finely sliced

1 small green pepper, finely
    sliced into rings
1 tablespoon chopped parsley
175 g/6 oz frozen sweet corn
1 quantity Short Crust Pastry
    (page 112)

Wash the fish and place it in a saucepan. Cover with water and season with a little salt and a bouquet garni. Cover, bring to the boil, and simmer very gently for 10 minutes or until the fish flakes easily. Remove the fish from the liquid, discard all skin and bones and flake the fish.

Heat the oil in a frying pan, add the garlic, the onion and green pepper and cook until soft. Add the parsley and season with a little salt. Grease a 1.15-litre/2-pint pie dish and layer the fish, sautéed vegetables and sweet corn in it.

Cover with short crust pastry and bake in a moderately hot oven (200c, 400f, gas 6) for 30–35 minutes until the pastry is golden brown. SERVES 4.

FRIED FILLETS OF SOLE

pinch of salt
4 tablespoons plain flour
4 large sole fillets
50 g/2 oz margarine

1 tablespoon oil
1 tablespoon chopped fresh dill
 or $\frac{1}{2}$ teaspoon dried dill

Add a little salt to the flour and dredge the fish fillets until evenly but lightly covered. Melt half the margarine with the oil in a frying pan and gently fry the fillets until golden brown on each side. Drain on absorbent kitchen paper and keep warm.

Wipe out the pan with kitchen paper and melt the other half of the margarine. When foaming, add the dill leaves. Cook for no more than 30 seconds, and then pour the flavoured margarine over the fish. Serve immediately. SERVES 4.

BAKED FILLETS OF SOLE

25 g/1 oz margarine
2 tablespoons fresh breadcrumbs
1 tablespoon chopped parsley
$\frac{1}{4}$ teaspoon dried mixed herbs
salt

nutmeg
4 large sole fillets
2 tablespoons browned
 breadcrumbs
a little extra margarine

Melt the margarine in a saucepan. Remove from the heat and add the fresh breadcrumbs, parsley and dried herbs. Season with salt and a little nutmeg and mix well.

Skin the sole fillets and spread the skinned side with the breadcrumb and herb mixture. Fold the fillets in half to enclose the stuffing.

Grease an ovenproof dish and put in the folded fish fillets. Sprinkle the fish with browned breadcrumbs and dot with a little margarine. Bake in a moderately hot oven (190 C, 375 F, gas 5) for 30 minutes until the topping is crunchy and the fish cooked so that it flakes easily. SERVES 4.

POACHED SALMON

trimmings from the salmon
1 parsley sprig
1 thyme sprig
1 small onion, chopped
1 carrot, chopped
1 bay leaf

salt
1.15 litres/2 pints water
1 tablespoon olive oil
1 kg/2 lb middle-cut fresh
   salmon

Place the first eight ingredients in a large saucepan to make a court-bouillon. Bring to the boil, cover and simmer for 30 minutes.

Add the oil to the bouillon and gently lower in the salmon in one piece. Cover the pan and poach carefully for 35 minutes. Do not let the fish boil rapidly as this will break the flesh. When the fish is cooked it will be bright pink and will flake easily.

To serve hot, remove the fish from the bouillon. Remove the skin and place the fish on a heated serving dish. Use the court-bouillon to make a parsley sauce (page 121). Serve with new potatoes and fresh peas.

To serve cold, allow the fish to cool in the court-bouillon, and then carefully remove and drain. Take off the skin and garnish the fish with cucumber slices. Chill in a refrigerator until needed. Serve with a green salad. SERVES 6.

BAKED SEA BREAM

1 large bream (about 1 kg/2 lb)
4 tablespoons oil
1 onion, chopped
100 g/4 oz fresh breadcrumbs

1 tablespoon chopped fresh
   parsley
1 teaspoon chopped fresh thyme
salt

Ask the fishmonger to clean and scale the bream.

Heat one tablespoon of the oil in a small saucepan and fry the onion until soft and transparent, but not brown. Stir in the fresh breadcrumbs and the chopped herbs and season lightly with salt. Fill the cavity of the bream with the stuffing mixture.

Grease a large ovenproof dish and place the whole fish in it. Sprinkle with salt and pour the remaining oil over. Bake in a moderately hot oven (190c, 375f, gas 5) for 45 minutes, basting frequently, until the fish is cooked and will flake easily, and the skin is crisp and golden brown. Serve immediately. SERVES 4.

PARCELLED MULLET

(Illustrated on page 52)

4 (175-g/6-oz) red or grey
  mullet
4 small rosemary sprigs
4 bay leaves
4 sage leaves

50 g/2 oz margarine
100 g/4 oz mushrooms, sliced
salt
4 tablespoons white wine
  (optional)

Ask the fishmonger to clean and scale the mullet.

Stuff each fish with a sprig of each of the herbs and a little margarine. Use the margarine to grease four pieces of foil, large enough to enclose each fish.

Place the fish on the foil and cover with mushrooms. Sprinkle with a little salt and pour over the wine, if used. Parcel up the fish and seal well so that none of the juices escape.

Bake in a moderately hot oven (190c, 375f, gas 5) for 25 minutes.
SERVES 4.

MACKEREL WITH CUCUMBER

4 mackerel, gutted
75 g/3 oz margarine
1 small cucumber, sliced

salt
2 tablespoons dry white wine
chopped fennel leaves to garnish

Remove the heads from the fish.

Grease a large shallow ovenproof dish with 25 g/1 oz of the margarine. Use half of the cucumber slices to cover the base of the dish. Place the mackerel on top of the cucumber and cover with the remaining slices. Season with a little salt, pour in the wine and dot with another 25 g/1 oz of the margarine. Cover the dish with foil or a lid, and bake in a moderately hot oven (200c, 400f, gas 6) for 30 minutes.

When cooked, arrange the fish and the cucumber on a serving dish and keep warm. Strain the juices from the fish into a small saucepan, bring to the boil and boil rapidly, adding the final 25 g/1 oz of margarine a little at a time. When the liquid has reduced by half pour it over the mackerel. Garnish with fresh fennel leaves and serve immediately. SERVES 4.

GRILLED MACKEREL FILLETS

allow 1 medium mackerel per person (about 350 g/12 oz each)

15 g/½ oz margarine or a little oil
parsley sprigs to garnish

Ask your fishmonger to fillet the mackerel.

Melt the margarine and brush both sides of the mackerel fillets with the fat. Oil can be used in place of the margarine if preferred.

Heat the grill and line the grill pan with foil, shiny side down. Grill the fillets, flesh side up, for 5 minutes. Turn the fish over and grill the skin side for a further 5 minutes. Finally turn the fish over again and grill the flesh side for a further 3–5 minutes until golden brown.

Place the fish on a heated serving plate and pour over the fish juices from the foil-lined grill pan. Garnish with parsley and serve immediately.

Note: This grilled mackerel is also delicious when cooled. Allow the fish to cool in its cooking juices, then serve the fillets with crisp toast. If the fish is served hot, then any which is left over can be reserved, cut into strips and served on toast for a quick, tasty snack.

HERRINGS IN OATMEAL

4 small even-sized herrings
salt
100 g/4 oz medium oatmeal

50 g/2 oz margarine
1 tablespoon corn oil

Cut the heads from the fish and split along the stomach. Clean the fish thoroughly. Open out the fish, place cut side down on a board and spread flat. Run your hand along the length of the fish, pressing firmly. Do this several times to press the bones away from the fish. Turn the fish over and pull off the loosened backbone. Remove as many bones as possible, and trim off the fins.

Sprinkle the fish, inside and out, with salt and coat with the oatmeal. Melt the margarine and oil in a frying pan, add the fish and fry gently for about 5 minutes each side until cooked through and golden brown. Drain on absorbent kitchen paper and serve really hot. SERVES 4.

Note: Mackerel can be cooked in the same way.

STUFFED HERRINGS

4 fresh herrings, cleaned
50 g/2 oz shrimps, chopped
1 tablespoon fresh breadcrumbs
1 anchovy fillet, mashed

salt
1 egg white, beaten
50 g/2 oz dry breadcrumbs
25 g/1 oz margarine

Remove the heads and fins from the herrings. Flatten out the fish, cut side down, on a board. Using firm pressure, rub the flat of your hand up and down the skin side of the backbone to press it away from the flesh. Turn the fish over and pull off the backbone and as many other small bones as possible.

Mix the shrimps with the fresh breadcrumbs and the anchovy fillet. Add a little water to moisten the mixture and a little salt. Spread a layer of the stuffing over the inside of the herrings and, starting at the head end, roll up the fish. Secure each with a metal skewer or wooden cocktail sticks.

Dip the fish rolls in the egg white and roll them in the dry breadcrumbs. Place them in a greased baking dish, dot with margarine, and bake in a moderately hot oven (190 c, 375 f, gas 5) for 30–35 minutes until golden brown. SERVES 4.

TROUT IN WINE

4 trout, cleaned
1 onion, sliced
100 g/4 oz mushrooms, sliced
150 ml/$\frac{1}{4}$ pint white wine
parsley sprig
2 bay leaves

thyme sprig
1 clove
blade of mace
salt
25 g/1 oz margarine
25 g/1 oz plain flour

Remove the heads from the cleaned trout. Place the fish in a shallow ovenproof dish and add the onion and mushrooms. Pour over the wine and add the herbs, spices and seasoning. Cover the dish and bake in a moderate oven (180 c, 350 f, gas 4) for 20 minutes.

Melt the margarine in a small pan and add the flour. Cook, stirring, for 2 minutes. Drain the liquid from the fish and transfer the trout to a heated serving dish. Strain the liquid and stir it into the margarine and flour, a little at a time. Bring to the boil and add a little more water if necessary to make a sauce with a pouring consistency.

Check the seasoning, and add a little salt if necessary. Pour the sauce over the trout and serve hot. SERVES 4.

TROUT AMANDINE

1 tablespoon plain flour
salt
4 trout, cleaned
75 g/3 oz margarine

1 tablespoon oil
50 g/2 oz flaked almonds
2 tablespoons chopped parsley

Season the flour with salt and use to coat the fish. Brush off the excess.

Melt half of the margarine and all the oil in a frying pan. Add the trout and cook for about 4–6 minutes on each side, until golden brown on the outside with white flesh. Do not overcook as this spoils the delicate flavour. Place the trout on a warm serving dish and keep hot.

Wipe out the frying pan with absorbent kitchen paper, then add the other half of the margarine. When the margarine is foaming, add the flaked almonds and cook until golden brown. Sprinkle in the parsley and cook for a further few seconds.

Pour the mixture over the trout and serve immediately. SERVES 4.

STUFFED TROUT

1 onion, finely chopped
50 g/2 oz mushrooms, chopped
75 g/3 oz margarine
3 tablespoons fresh breadcrumbs
1 teaspoon dried mixed herbs

salt
4 trout, boned
a little plain flour seasoned with
    salt
1 tablespoon oil

Prepare the stuffing by frying the onion and mushrooms in 25 g/1 oz of the margarine. When really soft, stir in the breadcrumbs, mixed herbs and salt. Leave on one side to cool.

Fill the inside of the trout with the stuffing and then re-shape the fish. Roll the trout in the seasoned flour and brush off any excess.

Melt the remaining margarine and oil in a frying pan and, when foaming, fry the trout until golden brown on each side.

Drain on absorbent kitchen paper and serve hot, garnished with parsley. SERVES 4.

White Fish and Corn Pie (page 44) with Glazed Carrots (page 94);
Honey Dreams (page 111)

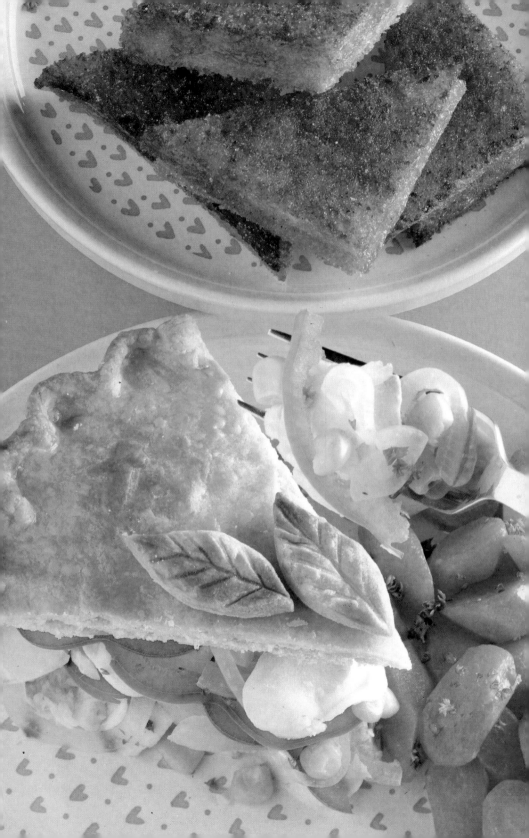

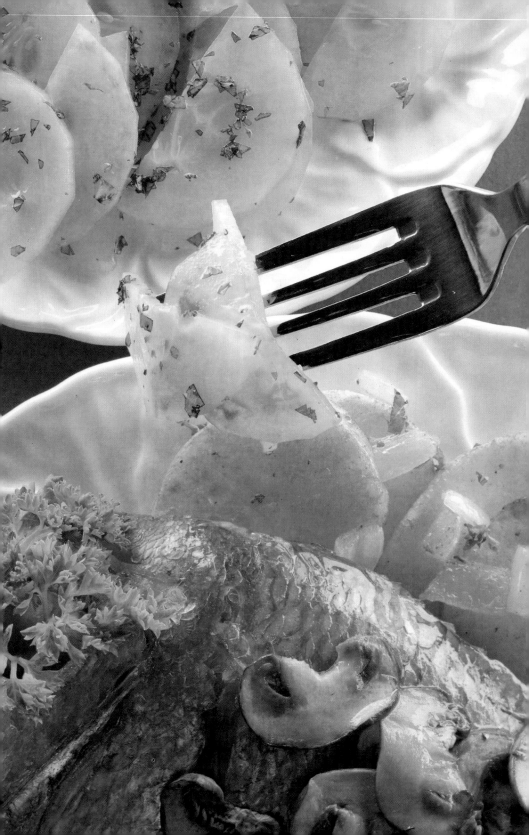

KEDGEREE

(Illustrated on page 33)

175 g/6 oz long-grain rice
175 g/6 oz smoked haddock
2 hard-boiled egg whites,
  chopped
1 tablespoon chopped fresh
  parsley

1 tablespoon chopped chives
salt
40 g/1½ oz margarine

Cook the rice according to the instructions on page 60 and fork up the grains so that they are all separate.

Heat a little water in a frying pan and, when boiling, put in the smoked haddock. Cover the pan and allow to simmer gently for 20 minutes until the fish is cooked and will flake easily. Drain the fish, remove all the skin and bone and flake the flesh.

Mix together the flaked haddock, cooked rice, hard-boiled egg whites and herbs, then season with a little salt. Melt the margarine in a saucepan and add the kedgeree. Stir gently over low heat until hot.

Serve with toast, for supper or breakfast. SERVES 4.

ARBROATH SMOKIES

allow 1 Arbroath smokie per
  person

margarine

Arbroath smokies are whole small haddock which have been smoked to a light brown colour.

Spread a little margarine over both sides of the smokies and grill for 4–5 minutes under a medium-hot grill, until the fish are heated through.

Serve with wholemeal bread and margarine.

*Parcelled Mullet (page 47) with Brialmont Potatoes (page 93)
and Cucumber Salad (page 100)*

FISH CROQUETTES

225 g/8 oz cooked white fish
225 g/8 oz cooked potatoes,
   mashed
1 tablespoon chopped fresh
   parsley
salt

nutmeg
a little plain flour
1 egg white
50 g/2 oz dry breadcrumbs
oil for frying

Flake the fish and mix it with the potato. Add the parsley and season well with salt and nutmeg. Mix and lightly chill the mixture.

Divide the mixture into eight. Shape each portion into a cork-shaped croquette or a round flat cake and coat each in flour. Dip the croquettes first in the egg white and then in the breadcrumbs. Press the coating on well. Fry the croquettes in oil until golden brown. Drain them on absorbent kitchen paper and serve hot. SERVES 4.

TUNA FISH FLAN

PASTRY
50 g/2 oz margarine
50 g/2 oz vegetable shortening
175 g/6 oz plain flour
2–3 tablespoons water

FILLING
1 (325-g/11-oz) can sweet corn

25 g/1 oz margarine
25 g/1 oz plain flour
1 (200-g/7-oz) can tuna fish
2 egg whites
6 anchovy fillets

Rub the margarine and shortening into the flour until the mixture resembles breadcrumbs. Add the water and mix to a dough.

Roll out the pastry and line a 20-cm/8-in flan ring. Prick it all over with a fork and place a piece of greaseproof paper in the flan. Put a handful of dried peas or beans on the paper to weight down the pastry. Bake in a moderately hot oven (190c, 375f, gas 5) for 10 minutes. Remove from the oven and take out the paper and dried peas.

To make the filling, drain and reserve the sweet corn and make up the liquid to 300 ml/½ pint with water. Melt the margarine in a pan, add the flour and cook until bubbling. Remove from the heat and gradually add the sweet corn liquid. Return to the heat and cook until thick. Add the tuna fish and sweet corn to the sauce and season it with a little salt.

Whisk the egg whites until stiff, then carefully fold them into the sauce using a metal spoon. Pile the mixture into the partly baked flan case and make a lattice of anchovy fillets on top. Bake for a further 30 minutes until the mixture is risen and golden brown. Serve either hot or cold with a selection of salads. SERVES 6.

MARY'S FRIED RICE

100 g/4 oz brown rice
salt
1 (99-g/3½-oz) can tuna fish
1 onion, chopped

1 clove garlic, crushed
100 g/4 oz sweet corn
1 teaspoon soy sauce

Cook the brown rice in salted water until just tender (see page 79).

Drain 2 tablespoons of the oil from the tuna fish into a large frying pan, add the onion and garlic and fry until soft but not brown. Drain the rice and add this to the frying pan, stirring the mixture so that the rice is well mixed with the oil and onion. Add the tuna fish and sweet corn and heat thoroughly. Stir in the soy sauce, mix well, and serve hot. SERVES 2–3.

TUNA POTATO PUFFS

1 onion, finely chopped
350 g/12 oz cooked potato,
     mashed
25 g/1 oz margarine

salt
nutmeg
1 (200-g/7-oz) can tuna fish
2 egg whites

Mix the onion with the mashed potato and the margarine, then season well with salt and nutmeg. Drain the oil from the fish, flake the flesh, and add it to the potato mixture. Whisk the egg whites until stiff and fold them into the potato mixture.

Grease the insides of four individual ovenproof dishes and pile in the mixture. Bake in a moderately hot oven (190c, 375F, gas 5) for 30 minutes and serve with Melba Toast (page 29). SERVES 4.

Main Dishes

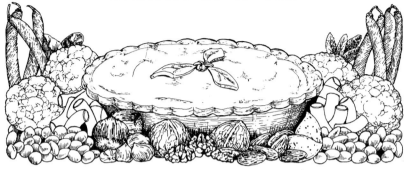

CHICKEN FRICASSÉE

4 chicken breasts
1 large onion, sliced
1 bay leaf
blade of mace
nutmeg
300 ml/½ pint water

300 ml/½ pint soya milk
50 g/2 oz margarine
40 g/1½ oz plain flour
salt
100 g/4 oz button mushrooms

Place the chicken breasts in a saucepan with the onion, bay leaf, blade of mace and some nutmeg. Mix together the water and soya milk and pour this over the chicken. Cover the pan, bring the liquid slowly to the boil, then reduce the heat and simmer carefully for 35 minutes.

Remove the chicken from the pan and cut the flesh into neat cubes. Place them in an ovenproof dish and keep warm. In a saucepan melt half of the margarine, then stir in the flour and cook for 2 minutes. Remove from the heat.

Strain the cooking liquid from the chicken and gradually pour this over the flour and margarine, stirring all the time. Return to the heat and cook until thickened. Season as necessary with a little salt, pour the sauce over the chicken and keep it hot.

Fry the button mushrooms in the remaining margarine until they are barely soft and sprinkle them over the fricassée. Serve immediately. SERVES 4.

ROAST CHICKEN

1.5-kg/3-lb roasting chicken
salt
2 rosemary sprigs
50 g/2 oz margarine

300 ml/$\frac{1}{2}$ pt chicken stock
150 ml/$\frac{1}{4}$ pt white wine
(optional)
2 teaspoons cornflour

Wipe the inside of the chicken, season it with salt, and place the sprigs of rosemary in the body cavity. Rub the margarine over the breast of the bird.

Place the chicken in a roasting tin and pour over the stock and wine. Roast in a moderately hot oven (190c, 375F, gas 5) for 1 hour, basting every 15 minutes. Transfer the chicken to a heated serving dish and keep hot.

Mix the cornflour with a little water; bring the liquid in the roasting tin to the boil and stir in the cornflour. Bring back to the boil, then simmer for 2 minutes, or longer if the gravy is too thin for your liking. If necessary, season with a little salt and serve separately. SERVES 4–6.

CHICKEN ANTONY

4 chicken breasts
1 tablespoon oil
50 g/2 oz margarine
1 clove garlic, crushed
1 onion, sliced
25 g/1 oz plain flour

300 ml/$\frac{1}{2}$ pint chicken stock
(page 21)
bouquet garni
salt
100 g/4 oz mushrooms, chopped

Sauté the chicken breasts in oil and half of the margarine until they are brown and sealed, then remove them from the pan.

Put the crushed garlic and sliced onion into the pan; brown them in the juices and oil and sprinkle in the flour. Cook for one minute and remove from the heat. Gradually add the chicken stock. Return to the heat and cook until thickened.

Replace the chicken in the pan and add the bouquet garni and salt to taste. Cover and simmer for 30–35 minutes. Meanwhile, melt the remaining margarine in a small pan and cook the mushrooms for about 2 minutes.

When the chicken is done, remove the bouquet garni and add the mushrooms to the sauce. Serve hot with mashed potatoes and a green vegetable. SERVES 4.

CERNEY CHICKEN CASSEROLE

4 chicken breasts
1 onion, chopped
1 carrot, chopped
bouquet garni
salt
50 g/2 oz margarine
50 g/2 oz plain flour
TOPPING
600 ml/1 pint stock from the
   chicken (above)

100 g/4 oz mushrooms
75 g/3 oz almonds
1 (340-g/12-oz) can asparagus
   spears
2 tablespoons oil
50 g/2 oz fresh breadcrumbs

Place the chicken breasts in a saucepan, cover with cold water and add the onion, carrot and bouquet garni. Season with a little salt. Cover the pan and bring to the boil. Simmer gently for 30 minutes. Remove the chicken breasts and strain the stock.

Melt the margarine in a saucepan and add the flour. Cook for 2 minutes, then remove from the heat. Gradually add the measured chicken stock. Return to the heat and cook until thick.

Cut the meat from the chicken breasts into neat pieces. Slice the mushrooms; blanch and split the almonds. Add the chicken, mushrooms and almonds to the sauce.

Place half the chicken mixture in a greased ovenproof casserole, and arrange the drained asparagus spears on top. Cover with the rest of the chicken mixture.

Heat the oil in a small saucepan and add the breadcrumbs. Fry until golden brown and sprinkle over the casserole.

Bake in a moderate oven (180c, 350f, gas 4) for 40 minutes. SERVES 4.

LEEKIE CHICKEN

salt
40 g/1½ oz wholemeal flour
4 chicken breasts
2 tablespoons oil

2 large leeks, cut into 5-mm/
¼-in slices
1 large carrot, sliced
450 ml/¾ pint chicken stock

Mix a little salt with the flour and use to coat the chicken pieces. Brush off any excess. Heat the oil in a saucepan and fry the chicken pieces until golden brown, but not completely cooked through. Remove the chicken from the pan and place on one side.

Add the vegetables to the pan and fry them over a low heat until soft. Sprinkle in the flour remaining from coating the chicken and cook this with the vegetables for 2 minutes. Remove from the heat and gradually stir in the chicken stock, then return to the heat and stir until the sauce boils and thickens.

Return the chicken pieces to the saucepan, stir well, then cover the pan and allow to simmer for 35 minutes. Stir two or three times during cooking to prevent sticking. SERVES 4.

CHICKEN IN WALNUT SAUCE

50 g/2 oz margarine
4 chicken breasts
150 ml/¼ pint white wine
2 tablespoons chicken stock
  (page 21) or water

50 g/2 oz walnuts, ground
salt
parsley

Heat the margarine in a frying pan and brown the chicken breasts on all sides. Pour over the wine and stock or water, cover the pan and simmer gently for about 25–30 minutes or until the chicken is tender. If the pan gets too dry, add a little extra water or stock.

When cooked place the chicken on a serving dish and keep hot. Bring the juices in the frying pan to the boil and add the ground walnuts. Add a pinch of salt and boil for 1–2 minutes. Pour the sauce over the chicken and garnish with chopped parsley. SERVES 4.

CHICKEN WITH CHESTNUTS

4 chicken breasts
3 tablespoons oil
1 onion, sliced
150 ml/¼ pint chicken stock
(page 21)

6 tablespoons soy sauce
6 tablespoons white wine
2 teaspoons caster sugar
1 (325-g/12-oz) can chestnuts

Cut each chicken breast into six pieces. Heat the oil in a frying pan and fry the onion for 2 minutes. Add the chicken and sauté for 6 minutes.

Add the stock and soy sauce. Cover the pan and simmer for 30 minutes, taking care that the liquid does not evaporate completely. Add the wine and sugar, stir well, and cook for a further 10 minutes. Stir in the drained chestnuts, and heat through.

Serve with plain boiled rice and a green salad. SERVES 4.

Note: Fresh chesnuts can be used in this recipe. Prepare them as described in Brussels Sprouts with Chestnuts on page 95, then cook them in stock or water for 15 minutes.

BOILED RICE

allow 40 g/1½ oz long-grain rice
per person

water
pinch of salt

Place the rice in a saucepan and rinse with several changes of cold water to remove excess starch. Drain well.

Level the rice in the bottom of the saucepan, and add enough water to double the depth of the rice. Add the salt, cover the pan tightly, then place it on a high heat and bring to the boil. As soon as the steam begins to escape, turn down the heat to very low. Leave to cook for exactly 12 minutes. Do not remove the lid during this time as it will allow the steam in which the rice is cooking to escape. At the end of 12 minutes remove the lid and fork up the rice to separate the grains.

Note: The smaller the pan you use for small quantities of rice, the better will be the result. Measuring the water correctly is most important, as too much means there will be water left in the pan at the end of the cooking time and too little will not cook the rice.

For parties, or when large amounts of rice are needed, cook the rice in 350 g/12 oz batches and allow each batch to cool. Pile on to ovenproof serving dishes, dot with margarine or sprinkle with a little oil and cover closely with foil. Reheat in a moderately hot oven (190c, 375f, gas 5) for 20 minutes. Fluff up with a fork and serve.

CHINESE FRIED CHICKEN

4 chicken breasts
6 tablespoons soy sauce
4 tablespoons white wine
½ teaspoon sugar

a little plain flour
oil for shallow frying
2 spring onions, chopped

Cut the chicken into bite-sized pieces and marinate it in the soy sauce, wine and sugar mixed together. Leave to stand for at least 1 hour.

Remove the meat from the marinade and dip each piece in flour. Heat a little oil in a frying pan and fry the pieces of meat until golden brown – this should take about 5 minutes. Heat the remaining marinade. Serve the chicken on a bed of plain boiled rice, garnished with spring onions and serve the marinade separately. SERVES 4.

CHICKEN MARYLAND

25 g/1 oz plain flour
salt
½ teaspoon dried oregano
4 boneless chicken breasts

2 egg whites
50 g/2 oz browned breadcrumbs
oil for shallow frying

Mix the flour with a pinch of salt and the oregano. Remove the skin from the chicken breasts, dip them in the seasoned flour and brush off any excess.

Lightly beat the egg whites and place the browned breadcrumbs on a flat plate. Dip the floured chicken first in the egg white and then in the breadcrumbs, pressing them on well to give a good coating.

Heat some oil in a frying pan and fry the chicken until it is cooked through. Start off over high heat to brown the meat and then reduce the heat and cook for 6–8 minutes each side.

Drain on absorbent kitchen paper and serve with Corn Fritters (page 97) and green vegetable or salad. SERVES 4.

SPICED CHICKEN

(Illustrated on back cover and page 69)

4 chicken breasts	75 g/3 oz margarine
1 onion, finely chopped	$\frac{1}{4}$ teaspoon turmeric
1 celery stick, finely chopped	generous pinch of cayenne
1 carrot, finely chopped	pepper
salt	$\frac{3}{4}$ teaspoon ginger
bouquet garni	$\frac{1}{4}$ teaspoon ground cumin

Place the chicken breasts in a pan. Cover with cold water and add all the vegetables. Season with a little salt and the bouquet garni. Cover the pan, bring to the boil, and simmer for 30 minutes. Allow the chicken to cool in the liquid.

Melt a third of the margarine in a small saucepan, add the spices and cook for 2–3 minutes. Allow to go cold.

Cream the rest of the margarine and beat in the cold spices. When the chicken is cold, remove from the liquid and place it on an ovenproof serving dish, spread over the spiced margarine, and chill.

Heat the grill and cook the chicken under it for about 6–8 minutes to brown the margarine. Serve the dish hot or cold with Rice and Prawn Salad (page 98). SERVES 4.

Note: This dish can be prepared well in advance of serving. Simmer the chicken, cool and spread with the spiced margarine, then cover and chill until required. This can be prepared a day or two in advance if you like, ready for grilling at the last moment.

CRUNCHY CHICKEN BAKE

75 g/3 oz margarine	4 chicken breasts
50 g/2 oz plain flour	100 g/4 oz mushrooms
300 ml/$\frac{1}{2}$ pint chicken stock	75 g/3 oz flaked almonds
(page 21)	salt
300 ml/$\frac{1}{2}$ pint soya milk	50 g/2 oz fresh breadcrumbs

Melt 50 g/2 oz of the margarine in a saucepan. Add the flour and cook for 2 minutes. Remove from the heat and gradually add the stock and soya milk mixed together. Bring the mixture to the boil and cook until thick.

Cut each chicken breast into four pieces and slice the mushrooms. Grease an ovenproof casserole and place the pieces of chicken breast and the sliced mushrooms in it. Sprinkle with the almonds and season with a little salt. Pour over the sauce.

Melt the remaining margarine in a small frying pan, add the fresh breadcrumbs, and fry until golden brown.

Sprinkle the crumbs over the casserole and bake in a moderately hot oven (200c, 400f, gas 6) for 40 minutes. SERVES 4.

Crunchy Chicken with Asparagus

For a special dish, asparagus can be substituted for the mushrooms in this recipe. Cook 225 g/8 oz asparagus, then lay the spears on top of the chicken. Sprinkle the almonds over and pour in the sauce. Continue as above.

MARINATED CHICKEN WITH ALMONDS

(Illustrated on page 34)

4 chicken breasts, boned
2 tablespoons soy sauce
1 tablespoon white wine
1 teaspoon ginger
2 tablespoons cornflour

4 tablespoons vegetable oil
100 g/4 oz blanched almonds, shredded
2–3 spring onions, chopped

Cut the chicken breasts into 2.5-cm/1-in squares and place them in a dish. Mix together the soy sauce, white wine and ginger, and pour this over the chicken. Mix well and allow to marinate for 1–2 hours.

Remove the chicken from the marinade and dust each piece with cornflour. Heat the oil in a frying pan and fry the pieces of chicken until golden brown and cooked through. Drain and pile them on a heated serving dish. Add the almonds to the oil and fry them until golden brown. Drain these and sprinkle them over the chicken.

Garnish with chopped spring onions. SERVES 4.

CHICKEN WITH BEAN SPROUTS

4 chicken breasts	450 g/1 lb bean sprouts
1 egg white	1 green pepper, thinly sliced
1 tablespoon cornflour	1 teaspoon sugar
salt	1 teaspoon soy sauce
4 tablespoons oil	

Cut the chicken breasts into long thin strips. Beat the egg white lightly and add the cornflour and salt. Place all the chicken in this mixture and mix well.

Heat 2 tablespoons of the oil in a large frying pan and add tablespoons of the chicken mixture to the pan. Stir around quickly to separate the pieces, then cook the chicken through. This should take 2–3 minutes if the chicken strips are thinly cut. Drain the chicken pieces on absorbent kitchen paper and keep them warm.

Add the remaining oil to the frying pan. Heat through and add the bean sprouts and the pepper. Cook for one minute, stirring all the time. Add salt to taste, sugar and the soy sauce. Stir in the chicken and mix it with the vegetables. Serve hot with plain boiled rice. SERVES 4.

SAGE CHICKEN BREASTS

4 boned chicken breasts	150 ml/$\frac{1}{4}$ pint dry white wine
a little plain flour	150 ml/$\frac{1}{4}$ pint chicken stock
salt	*(page 21)*
nutmeg	12 fresh sage leaves, coarsely
25 g/1 oz margarine	chopped
1 tablespoon corn oil	

Remove the skin from the chicken. Dip the chicken in the flour, which has been seasoned with salt and a little nutmeg.

Heat the margarine and oil in a frying pan and fry the chicken breasts until golden brown on both sides. Pour over the wine and stock and add the sage leaves. Cover the pan with a lid or plate and simmer the chicken for 20 minutes.

Remove the chicken and place on a heated serving dish to keep warm. Bring the remaining liquid in the frying pan to the boil and boil rapidly until reduced to about half the original quantity.

Strain the sauce over the chicken and serve hot with brown rice. SERVES 4.

TEXTURED VEGETABLE PROTEIN

Textured vegetable protein (TVP) is manufactured from soya beans to resemble either minced meat or chunks of meat. The dried products have to be soaked in stock or water before they can be cooked to make high-protein dishes. During soaking, TVP readily absorbs flavour fom herbs, spices, vegetables and stock, so it can be used in a wide variety of interesting dishes.

To reconstitute textured vegetable protein

Allow 25 g/1 oz of dry TVP per person. To soak the TVP, use chicken stock or yeast extract stock made by dissolving one teaspoon of yeast extract in each 300 ml/$\frac{1}{2}$ pint of boiling water. Allow 450 ml/1 pint of stock for each 100 g/4 oz of TVP.

Minimum soaking times for TVP

mince   5–6   minutes
flakes   15–20 minutes
chunks   25–30 minutes
large pieces   1–2   hours

These are minimum times – TVP can be left to soak for longer, even overnight.

CRUNCHY SOY

1 tablespoon yeast extract
300 ml/$\frac{1}{2}$ pint water

100 g/4 oz TVP slices
oil for frying

Dissolve the yeast extract in the water and pour this over the TVP slices. Allow to stand for 20–30 minutes or longer. Drain the slices and fry them in hot oil until golden brown. Drain on absorbent kitchen paper and serve.

These slices of TVP can also be soaked in chicken stock or vegetable juice and then fried as above. Serve as a snack with a Peanut Sauce (page 120) or as a main meal with Onion Sauce (page 120), potatoes and a green vegetable. SERVES 4.

TVP SLICES WITH GARLIC

2 teaspoons yeast extract
450 ml/¾ pint water
100 g/4 oz TVP slices
50 g/2 oz wholemeal flour
1 teaspoon dried thyme

2 tablespoons oil
2 tablespoons chopped fresh
  parsley
1 clove garlic, crushed
1 tablespoon soy sauce

Dissolve the yeast extract in the water and pour this over the TVP slices. Leave to soak for 2–3 hours or overnight. Drain the slices and reserve the liquid.

Mix together the flour and thyme. Heat the oil in a frying pan. Dip the TVP slices in the flour, fry in the oil until golden brown and place them in a casserole. Sprinkle each layer of slices with parsley.

Fry the garlic in the oil remaining in the frying pan and then add any remaining flour. Cook, stirring, until browned. Remove from the heat and stir in the reserved liquid, a little at a time. Return to the heat and cook until thick. Add the soy sauce and pour the sauce over the slices in the casserole. Cover the casserole and cook in a moderately hot oven (190c, 375f, gas 5) for 1½ hours. SERVES 4.

TVP HOTPOT

1 teaspoon yeast extract
1.15 litres/2 pints warm water
100 g/4 oz TVP chunks
1 tablespoon oil
2 large carrots, chopped
1 leek, chopped

1 large onion, chopped
2 celery sticks, chopped
50 g/2 oz long-grain rice
salt
1 teaspoon soy sauce

Dissolve the yeast extract in the water and pour this over the TVP. Leave to soak for one hour or longer.

Heat the oil in a heavy-based saucepan, and fry the prepared vegetables until they are golden brown. Add the rice and cook for a further 3 minutes.

Strain and reserve the liquid from the TVP. Add the chunks to the vegetables and cook for a few moments. Add the liquid left from the soaked TVP, and season the hotpot with salt and the soy sauce.

Bring to the boil, then cover and simmer for one hour on top of the cooker. Alternatively, transfer the hotpot to an ovenproof casserole and cook in a moderate oven (180c, 350f, gas 4) for 1½ hours.

Serve with Herb Dumplings (opposite). SERVES 4.

HERB DUMPLINGS

100 g/4 oz plain flour
salt
1 teaspoon baking powder

50 g/2 oz margarine
1 teaspoon dried mixed herbs
3 tablespoons water

Sift the flour with the salt and baking powder. Rub the margarine into the flour until the mixture resembles fine breadcrumbs. Mix in the herbs and add the water to make a soft dough.

Remove the lid from the casserole or saucepan in which the hotpot is being cooked and, 30 minutes before the end of the cooking time, drop small balls of the mixture on top of the vegetables. Replace the lid and continue cooking.

CHUNKY STEW

(Illustrated on page 70)

100 g/4 oz TVP chunks
1 teaspoon yeast extract
600 ml/1 pint water
1 tablespoon oil
1 medium onion, sliced
2 medium carrots, sliced

50 g/2 oz mushrooms, sliced
1 clove garlic, crushed
2 tablespoons plain flour
$\frac{1}{2}$ teaspoon dried oregano
salt to taste

Place the TVP chunks in a bowl. Dissolve the yeast extract in the water and pour this over the chunks. Allow to stand for 2–3 hours or overnight.

Heat the oil in a pan, add the vegetables and garlic, then fry for 10 minutes, or until the vegetables are golden brown. Drain the TVP and reserve the liquid, then add the chunks to the vegetables in the pan and fry for another five minutes. Stir in the flour and cook for a further two minutes. Remove from the heat and add the liquid from the soaked TVP, a little at a time, stirring between each addition.

Return the pan to the heat and stir until thickened. Lower the heat, sprinkle in the oregano and a little salt to taste, then simmer for 20 minutes. Serve with potatoes and a green vegetable or salad. SERVES 4.

MOUSSAKA

2 large aubergines *or* 1 large
    aubergine and 1 large potato,
    sliced
salt
2 teaspoons yeast extract
600 ml/1 pint water
100 g/4 oz TVP mince
oil for shallow frying
2 onions, chopped

100 g/4 oz mushrooms, chopped
1 clove garlic, crushed
2 tablespoons chopped parsley
SAUCE
25 g/1 oz margarine
25 g/1 oz plain flour
300 ml/½ pint soya milk
nutmeg

Sprinkle the aubergine slices with salt and leave on one side for 30 minutes. Dissolve the yeast extract in the water and pour this over the TVP mince. Leave to soak for 10 minutes or longer.

Heat the oil for shallow frying in a pan and fry the onions, mushrooms and garlic until soft and browned. Add the drained TVP and cook for two more minutes. Pour in sufficient of the yeast extract stock to just cover the contents of the saucepan, add the parsley, and season with salt. Cover and simmer for 10 minutes. Drain the aubergines and pat the slices dry on absorbent kitchen paper. Fry the aubergine and potato slices in a little oil until golden brown.

To make the sauce, melt the margarine in a small pan and stir in the flour. Cook for 2 minutes and remove from the heat. Stir in the soya milk, return to the heat, and cook until thick. Season with salt and grated nutmeg.

Grease an ovenproof casserole and place a third of the aubergine in the bottom. Cover with a layer of half the TVP mixture and cover that with another third of the aubergine. Add the rest of the TVP mixture, and finally cover this with the last of the aubergine. Pour over the sauce, dot the top with a little margarine and bake in a moderately hot oven (190c, 375f, gas 5) for 40 minutes. Serve with a Green Salad (page 99). SERVES 4–6.

Spiced Chicken (page 62) on Rice and Prawn Salad (page 98);
Carob Bavarois (page 109)

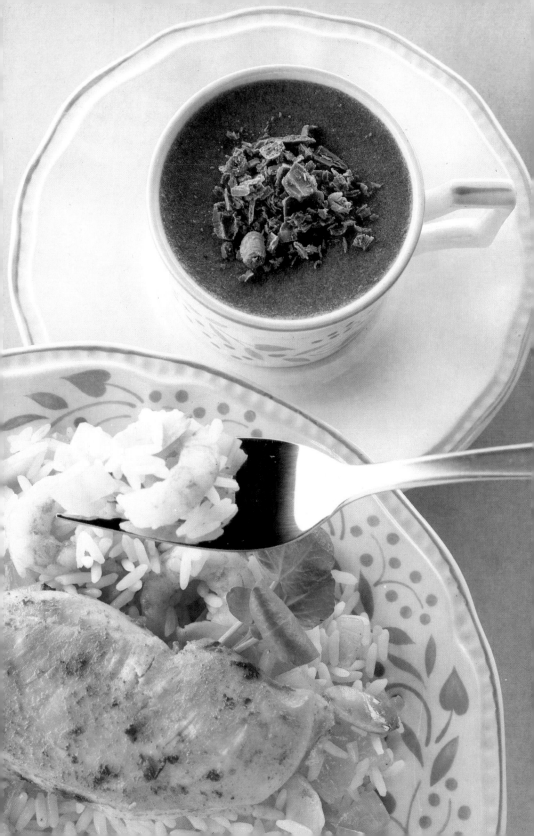

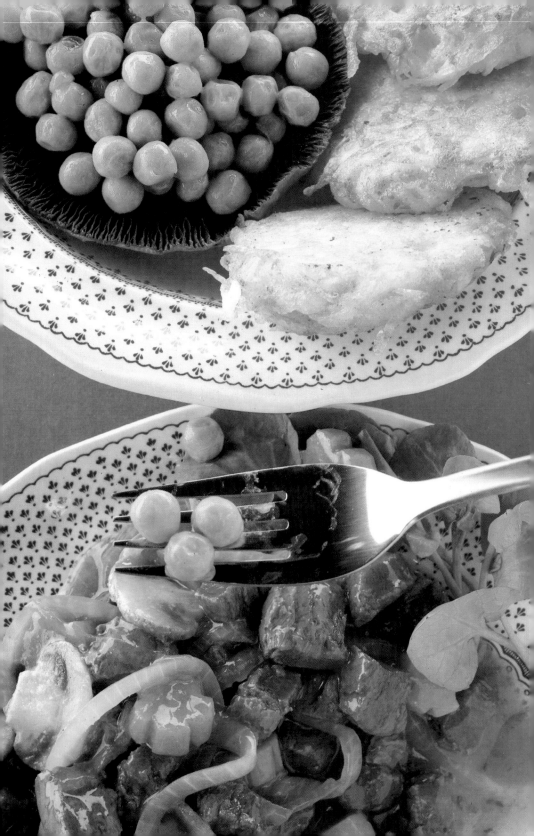

HARVEST PIE

PASTRY
175 g/6 oz wholemeal flour
50 g/2 oz soya flour
100 g/4 oz margarine
about 2 tablespoons water
FILLING
100 g/4 oz TVP flakes or chunks
600 ml/1 pint chicken stock
    (page 21)

2 medium onions, sliced
2 tablespoons corn oil
225 g/8 oz mushrooms, sliced
1 tablespoon cornflour
3 teaspoons water
salt

To make the pastry mix together the flours and rub in the margarine until the mixture resembles breadcrumbs. Add the cold water and mix the pastry until a soft dough is formed. Knead lightly. As this pastry is very short and crumbly, it is best to leave it covered in a refrigerator for about 30 minutes before rolling out.

Soak the TVP in the chicken stock for at least 20 minutes. Meanwhile, fry the onions in the corn oil until soft, add the sliced mushrooms and cook for a further 4 minutes. Drain the stock from the TVP and reserve this liquid. Add the drained TVP to the onion mixture and cook for 5 minutes. Pour over sufficient of the reserved stock to barely cover the TVP and vegetables.

Mix together the cornflour and water and add this to the pan. Bring to the boil, stirring all the time, to thicken the mixture. Season with a little salt, cover and simmer for 5 minutes. Pour the mixture into a 1.15-litre/2-pint pie dish. Allow to cool.

Cover with the pastry and bake in a moderately hot oven (200c, 400f, gas 6) for 30 minutes. SERVES 4.

Chunky Stew made with textured vegetable protein (page 67),
Mushrooms with Peas (page 95) and German Potato Cakes (page 93)

SINGAPORE SPECIAL

3 tablespoons soy sauce
3 tablespoons peanut oil
1 large onion, finely chopped
1 tablespoon grated fresh ginger
  root *or* 1 teaspoon ground
  ginger

6 coriander seeds, crushed
pinch of cumin
pinch of curry powder

Mix all the ingredients together. Dip slices of soaked TVP in the mixture before deep frying to make crunchy soy or use to brush over chicken breasts before grilling.

Note: The above mixture is sufficient to coat 100 g/4 oz TVP.

COUNTRY CASSEROLE

2 teaspoons yeast extract
600 ml/1 pint water
100 g/4 oz TVP chunks
50 g/2 oz lentils
3 tablespoons oil
1 large onion, sliced

1 clove garlic, crushed
1 red pepper, sliced
1 green pepper, sliced
2 tablespoons flour
bouquet garni

Dissolve the yeast extract in the water and pour this over the TVP chunks and lentils. Allow to soak for 30 minutes.

Heat 2 tablespoons of the oil in a frying pan and fry the onion and garlic until soft. Remove from the frying pan and place half the onion mixture in the bottom of an ovenproof casserole.

Drain the TVP and lentil mixture and reserve the stock in which they were soaked. Add the TVP and lentils to the frying pan and fry for 5 minutes. Layer the TVP and lentils, peppers and onions in the casserole, finishing with a layer of TVP and lentils.

Heat the remaining oil in the frying pan, add the flour and stir over the heat for 2 minutes. Remove from the heat and stir in the reserved stock, a little at a time, to make a smooth gravy. Pour this over the casserole, add the bouquet garni, cover and cook in a moderate oven (160 c, 325 F, gas 3) for 2½–3 hours. SERVES 4.

CROFTER'S PIE

1 teaspoon yeast extract
300 ml/½ pint boiling water
100 g/4 oz TVP mince
450 g/1 lb potatoes
1 large onion, chopped
1 clove garlic, crushed (optional)

1 tablespoon oil
1 tablespoon parsley, chopped
1 tablespoon chives, chopped
pinch of thyme
salt
a little margarine

Dissolve the yeast extract in the boiling water and pour this over the TVP mince. Leave until needed. Boil the potatoes until tender; drain and mash.

Fry the onion and garlic (if used) in the oil until soft and browned, and add the soaked TVP mince. Add the herbs and salt and mix well.

Pour this mixture into a pie dish and cover with mashed potatoes. Dot the top with a little margarine and bake in a moderate oven (180C, 350F, gas 4) for 30–40 minutes until the top is golden brown. SERVES 4.

TVP RISSOLES

1 teaspoon yeast extract
150 ml/¼ pint water
100 g/4 oz TVP mince
450 g/1 lb potatoes
1 medium onion, finely chopped

1 clove garlic, crushed
1 teaspoon dried mixed herbs
salt
50 g/2 oz plain flour
oil for shallow frying

Dissolve the yeast extract in the water and pour this over the TVP mince, then set on one side until needed.

Cook the potatoes in boiling, salted water until tender. Mash the potatoes and place them in a large mixing bowl. Drain the TVP and add this to the potatoes with the onion. Add the garlic and herbs and season lightly with a little salt. Mix thoroughly.

Divide the mixture into eight and shape each portion into a round about 7.5 cm/3 in. in diameter. Dip the rissoles in the flour and brush off any excess. Fry them in hot oil for 3 minutes each side until golden brown. Drain on absorbent kitchen paper and serve with a sauce (for example, Onion Sauce, page 120) made from any liquid left over from soaking the TVP. SERVES 4.

TVP PATTIES

2 teaspoons yeast extract
150 ml/¼ pint boiling water
100 g/4 oz TVP mince
50 g/2 oz fresh breadcrumbs

salt
1 teaspoon dried mixed herbs
1–2 egg whites
25 g/1 oz plain flour

Dissolve the yeast extract in the measured quantity of boiling water and pour this over the TVP mince. Allow to stand for 5–10 minutes.

Place the mince in a bowl and stir in the breadcrumbs, salt, and mixed herbs. Add enough egg white to bind the mixture together. Shape the mixture firmly into 4 round flat cakes.

Dip the shaped patties in flour, brush off any excess, and fry them in hot oil for 3–4 minutes each side. Drain on absorbent kitchen paper and serve hot. Serve as a main meal with a green vegetable, potatoes, and a sauce or gravy, or as a snack with salad. The patties may be used as a filling for a bread roll.

SPAGHETTI TEVENAISE

2 teaspoons yeast extract
300 ml/½ pint water
100 g/4 oz TVP mince
25 g/1 oz margarine
1 tablespoon oil
2 onions, finely chopped

2 carrots, finely chopped
100 g/4 oz mushrooms, chopped
a little white wine (optional)
salt
1 bay leaf
350 g/12 oz spaghetti

Dissolve the yeast extract in the water and pour this over the TVP mince. Leave to soak for 10 minutes or longer.

Heat the margarine and oil together in a saucepan and add all the vegetables. Fry until the vegetables are soft and golden brown.

Drain and reserve the stock from the TVP mince and add the mince to the vegetables. Fry for a further 5 minutes, then add sufficient of the liquid from the soaked TVP to just cover the contents of the saucepan. Add a little white wine, if used, season with salt and add a bay leaf. Cover the pan and simmer for 40 minutes until reduced and slightly thickened.

Meanwhile, bring a large pan of salted water to the boil and slowly add the spaghetti. Stir well and allow to cook for 12 minutes until the spaghetti is cooked, but still firm. Drain and pile the spaghetti on a heated serving dish. Pour the tevenaise sauce in the centre. Serve with a green salad. SERVES 3–4.

MACARONI SURPRISE

300 ml/½ pint soya milk
2 cloves
2 small onions
1 teaspoon yeast extract
300 ml/½ pint water
100 g/4 oz TVP mince
100 g/4 oz macaroni

salt
1 red pepper, finely chopped
1 tablespoon oil
1 tablespoon chopped fresh mint
25 g/1 oz margarine
25 g/1 oz plain flour

Place the soya milk in a small saucepan. Stick the cloves into one of the onions and place this in the milk. Bring to the boil, then leave on one side in a warm place.

Dissolve the yeast extract in the water and pour this over the TVP mince. Leave for 10 minutes. Meanwhile, cook the macaroni in boiling salted water until just cooked – about 12 minutes. Drain and leave until needed.

Chop the remaining onion and fry with the pepper in the oil. Drain the TVP mince and add this to the vegetables. Season with salt and mint, then cook slowly for 10 minutes.

Melt the margarine in a small saucepan and stir in the flour. Remove from the heat and add the strained, flavoured milk. Return to the heat and cook, stirring, until thickened.

Grease an ovenproof casserole and place half the macaroni in the bottom. Cover with half the sauce, and pour in all the TVP mixture. Top this with the rest of the macaroni and, finally, cover with the rest of the sauce. Bake in a moderately hot oven (190c, 375f, gas 5) for about 30 minutes. Serve with salad and bread. SERVES 4.

Note: This dish can be layered in the casserole some time in advance and cooked when required. It also freezes very well.

SOYA BURGERS

100 g/4 oz soya beans
600 ml/1 pint water
salt
225 g/8 oz potatoes, cooked and
   mashed

1 teaspoon soy sauce
1 small onion, finely chopped
1 egg white
a little plain flour
oil for shallow frying

Soak the soya beans in the water overnight.

Place the soaked beans in a saucepan and add enough water to cover. Simmer the beans, covered, for 4 hours or until tender. This can be done in a pressure cooker (following the manufacturer's instructions) to save time. Drain the beans, sprinkle with a little salt and mash them coarsely.

Mix the mashed beans and potatoes, then season with the soy sauce and add the onion. Bind the mixture with the egg white and, with wet hands, shape into eight round flat cakes. Dip the rounds in flour and fry them in oil until golden brown and heated through.

Serve the soya burgers on their own for a snack lunch with Peanut Sauce (page 120), or serve them with vegetables and Onion Sauce (page 120) as a main meal.

Note: These burgers can be made in quantity and frozen, uncooked, until required.

SOYA BEAN HASH

100 g/4 oz soya beans
1 tablespoon oil
1 large onion, finely sliced
2 cloves garlic, crushed
   (optional)

25 g/1 oz plain flour
1 tablespoon soy sauce

Soak the soya beans in water to cover overnight, then cook them, covered, for 4 hours, adding just enough water to cover them. Keep the beans covered with water as they cook. Drain the beans and reserve the liquid. Make this liquid up to 300 ml/$\frac{1}{2}$ pint with cold water.

Heat the oil in a small pan and fry the onion and garlic (if used) until soft and transparent. Stir in the flour and cook for 2 minutes. Remove from the heat, then add the liquid from the soya beans, a little at a time, stirring all the time. Return the mixture to the heat and cook until thickened. Add the soya beans and soy sauce and simmer for 5 minutes.

Serve this dish as a main meal with rice or potatoes and a green vegetable or salad. SERVES 2–3.

Vegetable and Bean Hash
Add 100 g/4 oz carrots and 2 sticks of celery, both diced, to the onion and garlic. About 2 minutes before the end of the cooking time, stir in 100 g/4 oz sliced mushrooms.

Curried Soya Beans
Fry 2–4 teaspoons curry powder with the onion and garlic. Add 1 bay leaf, a broken cinnamon stick and 2 cloves, then cook for a few minutes before adding the flour. If you like, serve small bowls of chopped hard-boiled egg white sprinkled with chopped onions, chopped cucumber and roughly chopped fresh peanuts as accompaniments.

Note: Cooked soya beans will keep in a refrigerator for 4–5 days if they are placed in a covered plastic container.

LENTIL AND VEGETABLE HOTPOT

100 g/4 oz lentils
600 ml/1 pint water
1 bay leaf
1 small onion, chopped
1 clove garlic, crushed
2 tablespoons oil

1 large onion, sliced
1 small cauliflower
50 g/2 oz green beans
salt
1 tablespoon soy sauce (optional)

Soak the lentils overnight, then simmer them gently in the water with the bay leaf, the chopped onion and the garlic for about 20–30 minutes until tender. Drain.

Heat the oil in a pan and fry the sliced onion until soft and brown. Meanwhile, break the cauliflower into florets and cut the beans into 1-cm/$\frac{1}{2}$-in pieces, cook them both in boiling salted water until tender.

Mix the vegetables with the fried onions, then stir in the cooked lentils. Season with a little salt, if needed, and soy sauce, if liked. Serve hot. SERVES 4.

NUT CUTLETS

100 g/4 oz mixed nuts
225 g/8 oz potatoes
¼ teaspoon dried basil or sage
1 tablespoon chopped parsley
salt

1 egg white
50 g/2 oz fresh breadcrumbs
oil for shallow frying
flour

Grind the nuts or chop them finely. Cook the potatoes in boiling salted water until tender. Drain them and reserve the water to make the sauce. Mash the potatoes.

Mix together the potato, ground or chopped nuts, herbs and season with a little salt. Allow the mixture to cool, and form into cutlet shapes or into round flat cakes.

Lightly beat the egg white. Dip the shaped nut mixture into a little flour, then into the egg white and finally into the breadcrumbs. Press the coating on well and allow the coating to harden for about 10–15 minutes before frying.

Heat some oil in a frying pan and fry the cutlets until golden brown – about 3–4 minutes each side. Serve with Onion Sauce, made with the potato water (page 120). SERVES 2.

NUT RISSOLES

100 g/4 oz lentils
salt
100 g/4 oz mixed nuts, ground
1 onion, finely chopped
1 clove garlic, crushed
pinch of dried sage

1 tablespoon chopped parsley
1 egg white
50 g/2 oz fresh brown
    breadcrumbs
oil for shallow frying

Soak the lentils overnight. Drain and boil them in salted water to cover until tender – about 30 minutes. Drain the lentils and reserve the liquid.

Mash the lentils well and add the ground nuts. Add the onion, garlic, herbs and seasoning, then bind together with the egg plus a little of the reserved lentil liquid, if needed.

Shape into rissoles and roll them in the breadcrumbs. Fry in oil until golden brown. Drain on absorbent kitchen paper and serve hot. SERVES 4.

NUTTY RICE

100 g/4 oz long-grain rice
1 onion, chopped
1 clove garlic, crushed
2 tablespoons corn oil
1 green pepper, chopped

225 g/8 oz mushrooms, chopped
100 g/4 oz mixed nuts, coarsely
  chopped
1 tablespoon soy sauce
pinch of salt

Cook the rice according to the instructions on page 60. Cook the onion and garlic in the oil in a large frying pan until soft and golden brown. Add the green pepper and mushrooms and fry for 2 minutes.

Stir in the cooked rice and nuts, and cook for a further 5 minutes. Add the soy sauce and salt to taste. Serve immediately with a Green Salad (page 99). SERVES 2–3.

BROWN RICE

allow 40 g/1½ oz of rice per
  person

water
salt

Bring 600 ml/1 pint water and 1 teaspoon of salt to the boil for every 50 g/2 oz rice.

When the water is boiling, add the rice and stir with a fork. Boil for 25 minutes until the grains are soft and tender. Drain the rice and return it to the pan with a small amount of oil or margarine. Shake the pan over a moderate heat to dry and glaze the rice.

Vegetables and Salads

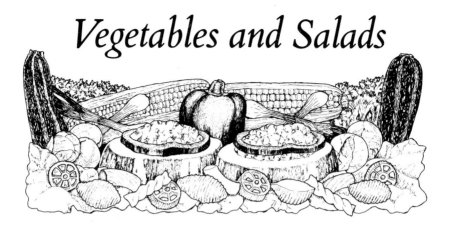

SWEET CORN SOUFFLÉ

1 (326-g/11½-oz) can sweet corn
50 g/2 oz margarine
50 g/2 oz plain flour

salt
nutmeg
4 egg whites

Heat the oven to moderate (180c, 350f, gas 4). Drain the liquid from the can of sweet corn and add enough water to make it up to 300 ml/ ½ pint.

Melt the margarine in a small pan, stir in the flour and cook for 2 minutes without browning. Remove from the heat and gradually add the sweet corn liquid, stirring all the time. Return the pan to the heat and cook until thick. Season with salt and a little grated nutmeg and add the sweet corn.

Grease a 15-cm/6-in soufflé dish. Whisk the egg whites until they are stiff and fold them into the sweet corn mixture. Pour the mixture into the soufflé dish and bake for 30–35 minutes until well risen and golden brown.

Serve immediately with a Green Salad (page 99). SERVES 2–3.

MUSHROOMS WITH RICE

4 tablespoons olive oil
1 onion, finely chopped
225 g/8 oz mushrooms, sliced
1 celery stick
2 tablespoons chopped fresh
parsley

150 ml/$\frac{1}{4}$ pint chicken stock
(page 21)
150 ml/$\frac{1}{4}$ pint white wine
salt
100 g/4 oz long-grain rice

Heat the oil in a saucepan and add the onion. Fry until the onion is golden brown then add the mushrooms. Stir well, cover the pan and cook for 3 minutes. Mix the celery into the mushroom mixture with the parsley, stock, wine and salt. Cover the pan and simmer gently for 15 minutes.

Stir in the rice and cook, covered, for a further 20 minutes or until the rice is cooked and all the liquid absorbed. Serve with a green salad. SERVES 2–4.

MUSHROOM CRUMBLE

75 g/3 oz wholemeal
breadcrumbs
175 g/6 oz mixed nuts, ground
1 clove garlic, crushed
1 teaspoon dried mixed herbs
100 ml/4 fl oz plus 1 tablespoon
oil

1 large onion, sliced
225 g/8 oz mushrooms, sliced
25 g/1 oz plain flour
150 ml/$\frac{1}{4}$ pint chicken stock
(page 21)
salt

Mix together the breadcrumbs, nuts, garlic and herbs. Pour over the 100 ml/4 fl oz oil and mix well. Leave on one side.

Heat the remaining tablespoon of oil in a frying pan and fry the onion until soft and brown. Add the mushrooms and cook for a few minutes more. Sprinkle in the flour and cook for two minutes. Remove from the heat and add the stock, stirring all the time. Return to the heat and cook until thick. Season to taste with a little salt. Pour this mixture into the bottom of an ovenproof casserole and sprinkle over the crumble mixture. Bake in a hot oven (220 c, 425 f, gas 7) for 30 minutes. Serve hot with vegetables and salad. SERVES 2.

MUSHROOM OMELETTE

2 egg whites
pinch of salt
1 teaspoon water

15 g/½ oz margarine
50 g/2 oz mushrooms, sliced
1 teaspoon oil

Break up the egg whites with a fork, add the salt and water. Melt the margarine in a frying pan and add the mushrooms. Cook for about 2 minutes, then remove them from the pan.

Place the oil in the pan and, when it is really hot, pour in the egg mixture. Stir it with a fork until it begins to set then leave to cook through.

Sprinkle the cooked mushrooms over half the omelette, fold the other half over and serve immediately. SERVES 1.

CHANGI MUSHROOMS

450 g/1 lb button mushrooms
BATTER
175 ml/6 fl oz tepid water
¼ teaspoon sugar
¼ teaspoon dried yeast
100 g/4 oz plain flour
1 egg white
SAUCE
1 celery stick, finely sliced
1 carrot, finely sliced
1 small red pepper, finely sliced

1 onion, finely sliced
1 tablespoon oil
300 ml/½ pint chicken stock
  (page 21)
1 tablespoon soy sauce
1 tablespoon cornflour
salt
oil for deep frying
chopped chives or spring
  onions to garnish

Remove and discard the stalks from the mushrooms (they can be used for soup). Wash and dry them and place on one side until needed.

Place the tepid water in a bowl and stir in the sugar. Sprinkle over the dried yeast and leave in a warm place for 5 minutes. Sift the flour into a bowl, make a well in the centre and add the yeast mixture. Stir until all the water and flour are mixed, then beat until the batter is smooth. Put in a warm place for 30 minutes.

Fry all the vegetables for the sauce in the tablespoon of oil for 2 minutes. Pour over the chicken stock and the soy sauce and bring to the boil. Mix together the cornflour and a little cold water. Add this to the sauce, stirring all the time, and cook until thick. If needed, season with salt, and keep warm.

Now return to the batter. Whisk the egg white until stiff and fold this into the batter. Dip the mushrooms in the batter and deep fry them until golden brown and puffy. Drain them on absorbent kitchen paper.

When ready to serve, pile the mushrooms on a heated dish and pour over the sauce. Garnish with chives or spring onions and serve with plain boiled rice. SERVES 4–6.

CABBAGE AND ALMOND BAKE

450 g/1 lb white cabbage, finely
  shredded
1 medium onion, finely sliced
salt
50 g/2 oz margarine
75 g/3 oz flaked almonds

25 g/1 oz flour
150 ml/¼ pint chicken stock
  (page 21) or soya milk
nutmeg
browned breadcrumbs

Cook the cabbage and onion in boiling, salted water until just tender – about 8–10 minutes. Drain and reserve the liquid.

Melt half the margarine in a frying pan and fry the almonds until golden brown. Sprinkle with salt. Heat the other 25 g/1 oz of margarine in a small saucepan and stir in the flour. Cook for one minute; remove from the heat and stir in the stock or soya milk and 150 ml/¼ pint of the cooking liquid from the cabbage. Return to the heat and cook, stirring, until thick. Season with salt and nutmeg.

Grease an ovenproof casserole with margarine or oil and place a layer of cooked cabbage in the bottom. Sprinkle most of the browned almonds on top and cover with half of the sauce. Repeat the layers and sprinkle with the browned breadcrumbs. Dot with margarine and bake in a moderately hot oven (200c, 400f, gas 6) for 15 minutes.

Serves 2–3 as a main dish, or 4 as a side dish.

FRIED CAULIFLOWER AND ONION

1 small cauliflower	oil for deep frying
salt	300 ml/½ pint batter *(page 122)*
1 large onion	

Break the cauliflower into florets and cook in boiling salted water for 10 minutes. Drain and leave on one side. Cut the onion into eight segments like an orange.

Heat the oil for deep frying to 180c/350f. Dip each piece of cauliflower in the prepared batter and fry in the hot oil until golden brown: this should take about two minutes.

Lower the heat slightly and dip the onion segments in the batter, then fry them for 4–5 minutes or until golden brown.

Drain the fried vegetables on absorbent kitchen paper, mix them together, and serve with salad and a Peanut Sauce (page 120). SERVES 2–4.

STUFFED PEPPERS

4 red or green peppers	salt
1 celery stick, finely chopped	½ teaspoon oregano
1 carrot, finely chopped	1 tablespoon soy sauce
100 g/4 oz mushrooms, chopped	50 g/2 oz flaked almonds
1 onion, finely chopped	150 ml/¼ pint chicken
2 tablespoons corn oil	stock *(page 21)* or water
100 g/4 oz long-grain rice	4 slices bread
1 tablespoon yeast extract	oil for shallow frying
300 ml/½ pint boiling water	

Cut the stalk end off the peppers and scoop out the white pith and seeds from the inside. Bring some water to the boil and blanch the peppers for 3 minutes. Drain them upside down. Chop away the pepper from around the stalk and mix it with the other vegetables.

Heat the oil in a saucepan, add all the vegetables, and cook them for 5 minutes. Stir in the uncooked rice and cook for a further 2 minutes.

Dissolve the yeast extract in the boiling water and add this to the rice. Season with a little salt, oregano, and soy sauce. Cover the pan and simmer for about 15 minutes until the rice is tender and all the liquid absorbed. Stir in the flaked almonds.

Stand the pepper cups in an oiled, shallow ovenproof dish and fill them with the rice mixture. Pour round the chicken stock or water, cover the peppers with a lid or foil and bake in a moderately hot oven (190c, 375f, gas 5) for 25–30 minutes until the peppers are tender.

Fry the slices of bread in a little oil until crisp and brown. Drain the peppers and place one pepper on each slice. SERVES 4.

STUFFED COURGETTES

50 g/2 oz lentils
1 bay leaf
1 onion, chopped
225 g/8 oz mushrooms, chopped
50 g/2 oz fresh breadcrumbs
3 tablespoons chopped parsley
1 teaspoon dried thyme

salt
1 egg white
8 small courgettes
300 ml/½ pint chicken stock
    (page 21)
1 tablespoon oil

Place the lentils in a pan of cold water and add a bay leaf. Cover the pan and simmer for 30 minutes, then drain.

Mix together the onion, mushrooms, breadcrumbs, herbs and cooked lentils. Season with a little salt and bind the mixture together with the egg white.

Peel the courgettes, cut in half lengthways and remove the seeds. Place them in a greased, ovenproof dish. Fill the centre of the courgettes with the stuffing and pour the chicken stock around them. Sprinkle the oil over and cover with foil. Bake in a moderately hot oven (190c, 375f, gas 5) for 25 minutes or until the courgettes are tender. Serve hot. SERVES 4.

Note: To thicken the sauce, pour off the chicken stock into a small saucepan. Mix 1 tablespoon cornflour with a little water and add to the stock. Bring to the boil to thicken the sauce. Season with a little soy sauce and pour over the courgettes before serving.

SPAGHETTI WITH AUBERGINES

1 large aubergine
salt
2 tablespoons oil
1 medium onion, chopped
1 clove garlic, crushed

1 red pepper, finely sliced
150 ml/$\frac{1}{4}$ pint vegetable or
  chicken stock
1 teaspoon oregano
225 g/8 oz spaghetti

Slice the aubergine into 5-mm/$\frac{1}{4}$-in slices, sprinkle with salt and allow to stand for 30 minutes. This will remove excess water and any bitter taste.

Heat the oil in a large frying pan and fry the onion and garlic until soft and slightly brown. Pour off the liquid from the aubergine and pat the slices dry on absorbent kitchen paper. Add the prepared aubergine and the pepper rings to the frying pan and cook until the vegetables are soft and well mixed. Pour over the stock, season with a little salt, and sprinkle over the oregano. Cover the pan and simmer for 15 minutes.

Cook the spaghetti in plenty of boiling salted water for 12 minutes until just cooked. Drain and toss in a little oil. Arrange the spaghetti on a heated serving dish and pour the vegetable mixture into the middle. SERVES 2.

Spaghetti with Aubergines and Chicory Salad (page 101)

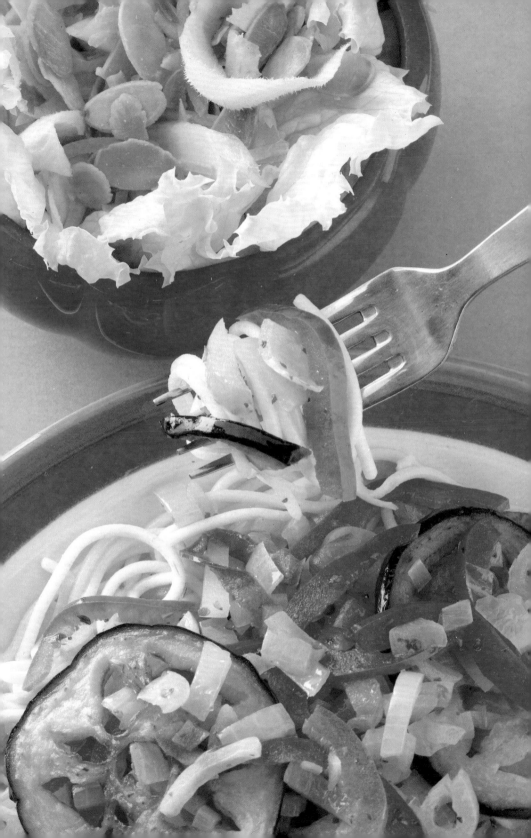

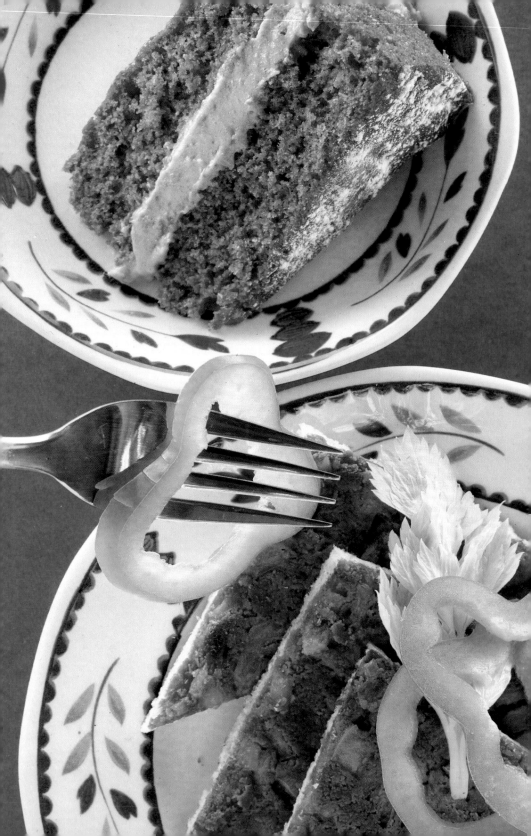

LEEKIE PIE

100 g/4 oz flaked TVP
600 ml/1 pint chicken stock *(page 21)*
3 large leeks
25 g/1 oz margarine
25 g/1 oz flour

salt
nutmeg
1 quantity Wholemeal Pastry
(page 113)

Soak the flaked TVP in well-flavoured chicken stock for 20 minutes or longer. Remove the root end from the leeks and cut off and discard the green top to within 2.5 cm/1 in of the white part. Cut the leeks into 2.5-cm/1-in slices and wash them thoroughly.

Grease a 1.15-litre/2-pint pie dish. Drain off any chicken stock that may be left unabsorbed and make it up to 300 ml/½ pint with water or extra chicken stock.

Layer the leeks and the TVP in the pie dish. In a small saucepan, melt the margarine, add the flour and cook for 2 minutes. Remove from the heat and add the chicken stock a little at a time, stirring well between each addition. Return to the heat and cook until thickened. Season the sauce with a little salt and grated nutmeg and pour it over the leeks and TVP in the pie dish.

Cover the pie with wholemeal pastry and bake in a moderately hot oven (200c, 400f, gas 6) for 30 minutes. Reduce the heat to moderate (180c, 350f, gas 4) and cook for a further 15 minutes. SERVES 4.

Note: You can use this recipe as a guide for preparing a mixed vegetable pie. Layer thinly sliced courgettes and lightly cooked sliced carrots with the TVP and leeks. Sliced green or red peppers, lightly fried in a little oil, and sliced cooked potatoes can also be added.

Irish Rarebit (page 103) and Portadown Cake (page 115)

STUFFED MARROW RINGS

1 medium marrow
2 tablespoons oil
1 small onion, chopped
225 g/8 oz mushrooms, chopped
175 g/6 oz wholemeal
    breadcrumbs

175 g/6 oz ground mixed nuts
1 tablespoon chopped parsley
salt
1 red pepper (optional)

Cut the marrow into 2.5-cm/1-in slices and carefully remove the centre seeds. Blanch the marrow rings in boiling salted water for 2 minutes only. Remove from the pan, drain and arrange the rings in a greased ovenproof dish in a single layer.

Heat the oil in a pan and fry the onion and mushrooms until soft. Add the breadcrumbs, mixed nuts and parsley. Season with a little salt and mix well. Spoon the mixture into the centre of the marrow rings and place a ring of red pepper on each slice. Bake in a moderate oven (180c, 350f, gas 4) for 20 minutes or until the marrow is tender.

Alternatively, the marrow can be sliced in half lengthways and, after scooping out the centre, blanched for 5 minutes before filling with the same mixture and baking in the same way. SERVES 4.

STUFFED ROAST ONIONS

4 large onions
salt
225 g/8 oz uncooked chicken
    breast, minced
a little plain flour

3 sage leaves, chopped
thyme sprig, chopped
parsley sprig, chopped
75 g/3 oz margarine

Peel and cut the root end off the onions. Large Spanish onions are good for this dish. Cook the whole onions in a pan of boiling salted water for 15 minutes. Drain the onions and, using a pointed knife, scoop out most of the inside.

Chop the scooped-out onion and mix it with the minced chicken. Spoon this stuffing back into the onion shells and press in well, taking care not to break the onions. Place them in a greased ovenproof dish; sprinkle with flour and the chopped herbs. Place a knob of margarine on each onion and roast in a moderate oven (180c, 350f, gas 4) for 40 minutes. Serve with plain boiled rice and a green salad. SERVES 4.

VEGETABLE CURRY

15 g/½ oz margarine
1 small onion, sliced
1 teaspoon curry powder
175–225 g/6–8 oz mixed cooked
  vegetables

50 ml/2 fl oz water
½ teaspoon yeast extract

Melt the margarine in a saucepan, add the onion, then cook until soft and golden brown. Stir in the curry powder and cook for a further two minutes.

Add the vegetables and pour in the water. Gradually stir in the yeast extract, making sure it is dissolved. Cover the pan and simmer for 10 minutes.

Serve the curry with plain boiled white or brown rice. SERVES 2.

ONION FLAN

175 g/6 oz plain white flour
salt
75 g/3 oz margarine
about 2 tablespoons cold water
FILLING
450 g/1 lb onions, finely sliced
1 tablespoon olive oil

12 black olives
1 (50-g/1¾-oz) can anchovy
  fillets
2 teaspoons chopped fresh or
  dried rosemary

Sift the flour and a pinch of salt into a bowl. Rub the margarine into the flour until the mixture resembles breadcrumbs and add sufficient water to make a dough. Leave in the refrigerator for 30 minutes.

Cook the onions in the olive oil until soft and golden brown. Allow to cool. Remove the stones from the olives. Drain the anchovies and keep the oil.

Roll out the pastry to line a 20-cm/8-in flan tin. Cover the base with the fried onions and make a lattice over the top with the anchovy fillets. Place a black olive in each square, and sprinkle the flan with rosemary. Pour over the oil from the can of anchovies and bake in the hot oven for 30–35 minutes. Serve warm. SERVES 4.

FLUFFY BAKED POTATOES

4 large old potatoes
50 g/2 oz margarine
1 small onion, finely chopped

$\frac{1}{2}$ teaspoon soy sauce
2 egg whites

Scrub the potatoes, prick them with a fork and bake for about $1\frac{1}{2}$ hours in a moderate oven (180C, 350F, gas 4). When the potatoes are cooked cut them in half and scoop the insides into a bowl. Mash the margarine into the potatoes and add the onion. Season with a little soy sauce to taste.

Whisk the egg whites until they are stiff then carefully fold them into the potatoes. Spoon the mixture in the potato skins and return them to the oven to cook for a further 15 minutes. SERVES 4.

POTATO PIE

450 g/1 lb potatoes
25 g/1 oz margarine
1 tablespoon chopped chives
225 g/8 oz cooked sweet corn

50 g/2 oz flaked almonds
1 small red or green pepper,
   diced

Cook the potatoes in boiling salted water until tender, then strain and mash well with the margarine and chives.

Grease a pie dish and place half the potato in the dish. Cover with a layer of sweet corn, almonds, and the red or green pepper. Cover with the rest of the potatoes. Fork the top into peaks and dot with margarine.

Bake in a moderately hot oven (190C, 375F, gas 5) for 30 minutes until the top is golden brown. Serve with a green salad. SERVES 2–3.

GERMAN POTATO CAKES

(Illustrated on page 70)

450 g / 1 lb even-sized potatoes	pinch of cinnamon
1 onion, grated	1 egg white
salt	little corn oil

Scrub the potatoes, place them in a saucepan and just cover with cold water. Bring to the boil, then reduce the heat and allow to simmer for just 7 minutes. Pour off the boiling water, cover with cold water, and leave the potatoes to cool. When cold, remove their skins and grate the potatoes.

Add the onion to the grated potatoes. Mix well, season with a little salt and a pinch of cinnamon, then stir in the egg white.

Heat a little corn oil in a frying pan and, when really hot, drop spoonfuls of the potato mixture into the pan. Flatten with a palette knife and, when set and golden underneath, turn over and cook the other side until golden brown. Serve with fish or chicken and salad. MAKES 20.

BRIALMONT POTATOES

(Illustrated on page 52)

450 g / 1 lb even-sized potatoes	2 tablespoons chopped parsley
50 g / 2 oz margarine	salt
1 onion, finely chopped	

Scrub the potatoes and cook them in their skins in boiling water for 15 minutes. Drain and allow to cool. Remove their skins and slice the potatoes into neat rounds about 5 mm / $\frac{1}{4}$ in thick.

Melt the margarine in a small frying pan. Add the onion and cook until soft but not brown. Add the parsley and season the mixture with salt to taste.

Layer the potatoes with the onion and parsley mixture in a greased ovenproof dish, finishing with a layer of the onion and parsley mixture on top. Cook, uncovered, in a moderately hot oven (190c, 375f, gas 5) for 20–30 minutes until the potatoes are soft and golden brown on top. SERVES 4.

GLAZED CARROTS

(Illustrated on page 51)

450 g/1 lb new or old carrots
2 teaspoons sugar
50 g/2 oz margarine

½ teaspoon salt
1 tablespoon chopped parsley

Peel or scrape the carrots, then slice and place them in a saucepan with just enough water to cover. Add the sugar, margarine and salt. Bring to the boil. Boil rapidly, uncovered, until the carrots are tender and all the water has evaporated. Sprinkle with chopped parsley and serve. SERVES 4.

MOULDED CAULIFLOWER

1 medium cauliflower
salt
25 g/1 oz margarine
1 small clove garlic, finely
  chopped

25 g/1 oz flaked almonds
3 tablespoons fresh breadcrumbs

Break the cauliflower into florets and cook in boiling salted water until tender – about 15 minutes. Drain the cooked cauliflower thoroughly to remove as much water as possible.

Grease the inside of a 1.15-litre/2-pint pudding basin with a little margarine and arrange the cauliflower sprigs in this. Try to keep the stalks to the centre of the basin. Cover with a plate and press down with a little gentle pressure to mould the cauliflower. Leave on one side to keep hot.

Melt the margarine in a small saucepan and fry the garlic. Add the flaked almonds and the breadcrumbs, stir well and cook until golden brown.

Turn the moulded cauliflower out on to a hot serving dish and spoon over the breadcrumb mixture. SERVES 4.

MUSHROOMS WITH PEAS

(Illustrated on page 70)

225 g/8 oz fresh peas
salt
½ teaspoon sugar
1 sprig mint

2 tablespoons chicken stock
50 g/2 oz margarine
8 large flat mushrooms

Cook the peas in boiling salted water with the sugar and mint for 15 minutes. Drain the peas, return them to the pan, and pour over the chicken stock. Add half the margarine. Cook, uncovered, until all the stock has been absorbed.

Wipe the mushrooms and remove the stalks (they can be used in soups or sauces). Melt the remaining margarine in a frying pan and carefully fry the mushrooms for 5 minutes. Place the mushroom caps on a serving dish and spoon the peas into them. Serve immediately. SERVES 4.

Note: This recipe can be made with frozen peas, but they should be cooked for just a minute.

BRUSSELS SPROUTS WITH CHESTNUTS

175 g/6 oz chestnuts
450 g/1 lb small Brussels sprouts
600 ml/1 pint chicken stock
    (page 21)

salt
25 g/1 oz margarine

First prepare the chestnuts. Make a small slit in the flat side of the nuts and place them in a baking tin. Place in a moderately hot oven (200c, 400f, gas 6) and bake for 10 minutes. During this time both layers of skin around the chestnuts will crack. Peel off the skin while the nuts are still warm.

Meanwhile, wash and trim the sprouts and make a small slit in the stem of each one. Bring the stock to the boil and season with salt if necessary. Add the sprouts and the chestnuts, bring back to the boil, then cover the pan and simmer for 20 minutes.

Drain off the stock. Melt the margarine in a saucepan, add the sprouts and chestnuts, and shake the pan over a moderate heat to glaze the vegetables and nuts. Serve immediately. SERVES 4.

MINTED PEAS

225 g/8 oz frozen peas
1 mint sprig
1 small onion, chopped

1 scant teaspoon sugar
salt
1 tablespoon water

Place the peas in a greased ovenproof dish. Add the mint, onion, sugar and a sprinkling of salt. Pour over the water and cover the dish with a lid or kitchen foil. Cook in a moderate oven (180c, 350f, gas 4) for 20 minutes. SERVES 2.

Note: These peas can also be cooked in a small saucepan on top of the cooker. The above cooking method is useful if you already have another dish in the oven.

VEGETABLE COCKTAIL

(Illustrated on page 33)

1 carrot, chopped
1 celery stick, chopped
1 tablespoon chopped fresh mint
$\frac{1}{4}$ teaspoon oregano

pinch of salt
1 teaspoon yeast extract
150 ml/$\frac{1}{4}$ pint hot water

Place the chopped vegetables in an electric blender. Add the herbs and salt. Dissolve the yeast extract in the water, then pour into the liquidiser. Blend until smooth and pour through a sieve to remove the stringy fibres from the celery. Serve chilled. SERVES 1.

Note: This cocktail is very rich in vitamins A and C.

CORN FRITTERS

100 g/4 oz plain flour
pinch of salt
2 teaspoons soya flour

2 egg whites
1 (325-g/12-oz) can sweet corn
corn oil for frying

Sift the flour, salt and soya flour together into a bowl, make a well in the centre and add the egg whites. Drain the sweet corn, reserving 4 tablespoons of the liquid from the can. Add 1 tablespoon of this liquid to the egg white. Mix to a smooth batter and beat well. Add the rest of the sweet corn liquid, and leave the batter to stand for 10 minutes.

Heat a little corn oil in a frying pan. Add the sweet corn to the batter and drop spoonfuls of the mixture into the hot oil. Fry the fritters on both sides until golden brown and puffy. Drain on absorbent kitchen paper and serve hot. SERVES 4.

SALMON PASTA SHELL SALAD

225 g/8 oz pasta shells
1 (213-g/7½-oz) can salmon or
  tuna fish
2 teaspoons chopped fresh
  mixed herbs *or* 1 teaspoon
  dried mixed herbs

3 tablespoons olive oil
salt
1 lettuce, shredded
cucumber slices to garnish

Bring a pan of salted water to the boil and pour in the pasta shells. Stir to prevent them sticking together, return to the boil and cook for 12 minutes until the pasta is just cooked but still firm. Drain and rinse the pasta shells under cold water. Transfer them to a bowl.

Drain the liquid from the salmon or tuna fish into a small bowl and add the herbs, olive oil and salt. Whisk the mixture throughly.

Mix together the flaked fish and the pasta shells and arrange them neatly on a bed of lettuce. Pour over the oil and herb mixture and garnish the dish with cucumber slices.

Serve cold with wholemeal bread. SERVES 4.

ANCHOVY SALAD

1 clove garlic, crushed
salt
3 tablespoons olive oil
1 (213-g/7½-oz) can tuna fish
1 red pepper

1 green pepper
1 lettuce
1 onion, finely sliced
1 (50-g/1¾-oz) can anchovies
12 black olives

Add the garlic with a little salt to the olive oil then add 1 tablespoon of the oil from the tuna fish.

Place the red and the green peppers under a hot grill and turn them frequently so that the skins become black and blistered. Hold the peppers under cold running water, to remove the skin. Cut off the stalk end, scoop out the seeds, and shred the flesh into slices.

Arrange the lettuce on a serving plate. Mix the drained tuna fish, peppers and onion. Pile on top of the lettuce. Arrange the anchovy fillets in a lattice pattern over the salad and place a black olive in each little square. Pour over the olive oil dressing and chill well before serving. SERVES 4.

RICE AND PRAWN SALAD

(Illustrated on page 69)

100 g/4 oz long-grain rice
1 small onion, finely chopped
15 g/½ oz margarine
100 g/4 oz cooked prawns

50 g/2 oz flaked almonds
2 tablespoons oil
salt

Cook the rice according to the instructions on page 60 and allow to go cold.

Fry the onion in the margarine until it is soft and transparent. In a salad bowl mix together the rice, onion, prawns, and the flaked almonds.

Whisk the oil with a little salt and pour this over the salad. Mix well and serve chilled. This salad is a very good accompaniment for Spiced Chicken (page 62). SERVES 4.

MUSHROOM AND PRAWN SALAD

225 g/8 oz mushrooms
100 g/4 oz peeled prawns or
   shrimps
4 tablespoons olive oil

salt
2 teaspoons chopped mixed
   fresh herbs
mustard and cress

Wash the mushrooms, slice them thinly and place on a flat dish. Sprinkle the prawns or shrimps over the mushrooms.

Mix the olive oil with the salt and the chopped herbs. If canned prawns or shrimps are used, add 1 tablespoon of the liquid from the can to the dressing. Whisk the dressing thoroughly, then pour it over the salad.

Allow the salad to stand in a cool place for one hour before serving. Garnish with mustard and cress and serve with brown bread and margarine.

GREEN SALAD

A green salad can be made of one or a mixture of any of the following salad vegetables:

lettuce
mustard and cress
watercress
chicory
endive
green peppers, finely sliced

DRESSING
1 clove garlic
olive or salad oil

Wash the chosen salad vegetables and dry them really well. Prepare them according to type.

Cut the clove of garlic in two and rub the cut side around the inside of a salad bowl. Put in the salad vegetables. Just before serving pour in just enough salad dressing to coat all the leaves of the salad. Toss well to make sure the dressing is well mixed. Serve immediately.

CUCUMBER SALAD

(Illustrated on page 52)

½ cucumber
1 teaspoon salt

1 tablespoon olive oil *or* salad oil
1 teaspoon chopped mint

Peel the cucumber, split it in half lengthways and then cut it into 5-mm/¼-in slices. Sprinkle with salt and allow to stand for 30 minutes. When the time is up, pour off the liquid from the cucumber and add this to the oil. Whisk this mixture and add the chopped mint. Pour the dressing over the cucumber and serve chilled. SERVES 2.

RICE AND NUT SLAW

½ small white cabbage, finely
  shredded
2 medium carrots, grated
1 green pepper, trimmed and
  finely shredded

225 g/8 oz cooked rice
3 tablespoons Creamy Salad
  Dressing *(page 121)*
lettuce leaves to serve
50 g/2 oz walnuts

Mix the prepared vegetables with the rice and add just enough dressing to moisten the mixture. Serve on a bed of lettuce, and sprinkle the nuts over. SERVES 4.

Note: This salad can be served as the main dish for a light lunch or as an accompaniment to a TVP dish.

POTATO SALAD

450 g/1 lb new potatoes
50 g/2 oz peas (frozen or fresh)
salt
1 teaspoon chopped parsley
1 teaspoon chopped onion

1 pinch of dried tarragon
Creamy Salad Dressing
  (page 121)
1 small lettuce, washed and
  shredded

Wash the potatoes and boil them in their skins until tender. Plunge them into cold water and remove the skins. Cut the peeled potatoes into neat dice.

Cook the peas in a little salted water; drain and allow to cool. Mix together the diced potatoes and cooked peas in a salad bowl, add the parsley, onion and tarragon and a little salt. Pour over enough dressing to moisten the potatoes then serve the salad on a bed of shredded lettuce. SERVES 2.

SPRING SALAD

175 g/6 oz cooked chicken breast, diced
½ small white cabbage, finely shredded
2 large carrots, grated
1 small onion, finely sliced

4 celery sticks, sliced thinly
salt
150 ml/¼ pint Creamy Salad Dressing *(page 121)*
50 g/2 oz peanuts

Mix the diced chicken with the vegetables and season lightly with salt. Pour over the dressing, toss lightly and sprinkle the peanuts on top.

Serve with potatoes baked in their jackets or crusty bread. SERVES 2–3.

CHICORY SALAD

(Illustrated on page 87)

4 heads of chicory
25 g/1 oz flaked almonds
a little oil
salt

4 large carrots, grated
150 ml/¼ pint Creamy Salad Dressing *(page 121)*
lettuce leaves to serve

Thinly slice the chicory. Fry the almonds in a little oil until golden brown; drain on absorbent kitchen paper and sprinkle with a little salt.

Mix the chicory and carrot then toss in the creamy dressing. Pile on to lettuce leaves and sprinkle over the almonds. SERVES 4.

Savouries and Snacks

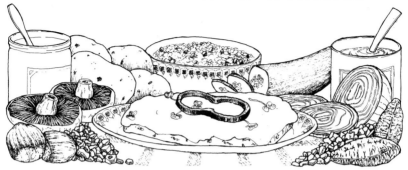

SALMON SAVOURIES

8 slices wholemeal bread
50 g/2 oz margarine
1 (99-g/3½-oz) can salmon or
   tuna fish

salt
2 egg whites
oil for shallow frying
sliced cucumber to garnish

Remove the crusts from the bread and spread each slice with margarine. Sandwich the slices together with the mashed salmon or tuna fish seasoned with a little salt. Cut each sandwich into four triangles.

Whisk the egg whites until just broken. Heat some oil in a frying pan. Dip the sandwiches in the egg white and fry them in the hot oil until crisp and golden brown. Drain on absorbent kitchen paper and serve garnished with sliced cucumber. SERVES 4.

FRENCH TOAST

2 slices bread
yeast extract
1 egg white

salt
oil for frying

Halve the slices of bread and spread with a little yeast extract. Lightly beat the egg white with a pinch of salt.

Heat a little oil in a frying pan. Dip the bread in the egg mixture and fry in the hot oil until golden brown. Drain on absorbent kitchen paper and serve hot. SERVES 1.

IRISH RAREBIT

(Illustrated on page 88)

40 g/1½ oz margarine
¼ teaspoon yeast extract
25 g/1 oz soya flour
1 tablespoon chopped onion

1 tablespoon chopped green
  pepper
2 slices toast

Melt the margarine in a small pan and add the yeast extract. Stir in the soya flour and cook the mixture until it bubbles. Add the onion and pepper and pile the mixture on to the toast. Place under a hot grill to cook the vegetables and slightly brown the mixture. SERVES 1.

MUSHROOMS ON TOAST

15 g/½ oz margarine *or*
  1 tablespoon oil
50 g/2 oz flat mushrooms

salt
1 slice wholemeal bread

Heat the margarine or oil in a frying pan and add the clean, dry mushrooms. Sprinkle them with a little salt and shake the pan to coat each of the mushrooms in a little fat. Lower the heat, cover the pan, and allow the mushrooms to cook until just soft (about 5–8 minutes).

Meanwhile, toast the bread and spread lightly with margarine. Pile the cooked mushrooms on the hot toast and serve immediately. SERVES 1.

IRISH EGGS

450 g/1 lb potatoes
25 g/1 oz margarine
salt
4 hard-boiled egg whites
1 teaspoon chopped chives

50 g/2 oz cooked lentils
2–4 tablespoons flour
1 egg white
browned breadcrumbs
oil for frying

Mash the potatoes with the margarine and season with a little salt, if necessary. Chop the cooked egg whites. Mix the chives with the potatoes and the lentils. Mix really well and shape into round cakes.

Dip them in a little flour, then in beaten egg white, and finally in browned breadcrumbs. Fry in oil until golden brown and drain on absorbent kitchen paper.

For quickness, these cakes can be dipped in flour and then fried.
SERVES 2–4.

FRIED RICE

100 g/4 oz long-grain rice
2 tablespoons oil
1 onion, chopped
25 g/1 oz margarine

175 g/6 oz frozen mixed
  vegetables
1 tablespoon soy sauce
pinch of curry powder

Cook the rice according to the instructions on page 60.

Heat the oil in a frying pan and fry the onion until soft and golden brown. Stir in the cooked rice, add the margarine and fry until the rice is really hot.

Cook the frozen vegetables according to the directions on the packet. Add the cooked vegetables to the rice mixture. Turn up the heat and stir in the soy sauce and the curry powder. Add a little salt if necessary. Serve with prawn crackers and Green Salad (page 99).
SERVES 2.

Prawn Fried Rice
Add 100 g 4 oz peeled prawns just before stirring in the cooked rice.

Fried Rice with Peppers
Trim and dice 1 red pepper and 1 green pepper. Cook these with the onion, then continue as above.

ANCHOVY SPREAD

1 (50-g/1¾-oz) can anchovies   50 g/2 oz margarine

Drain the oil from the anchovies and lightly rinse the fillets in water to reduce their saltiness. Drain and dry them on absorbent kitchen paper.

Pound the anchovy fillets in a pestle and mortar until a smooth paste is obtained. Alternatively, you can mash the fillets with a fork.

Cream the margarine until soft and beat in the anchovies. Chill and store in a cool place.

Serve with hot toast.

CAROB SPREAD

100 g/4 oz margarine   50 g/2 oz flaked almonds,
2 tablespoons golden syrup   broken
1 tablespoon carob powder

Cream the margarine and golden syrup until well mixed. Beat in the carob powder and stir in the flaked almonds.

Store in a jam jar in the refrigerator and serve spread on bread or toast.

MOUSSELI

1 tablespoon chopped mixed   pinch of ground mixed spice or
  nuts   cinnamon
2 tablespoons rolled oats   2 teaspoons brown sugar
2 teaspoons soya flour

Place the nuts in a bowl with the rolled oats. Sprinkle over the soya flour, spice and sugar, and mix well. Stir in enough water to make a thick mixture and serve immediately. SERVES 2.

FLUFFY OMELETTE

1 tablespoon soya flour
4 tablespoons water
1 teaspoon oil
2 egg whites

oil for frying
maple or golden syrup to
  serve

Place the soya flour in a small saucepan. Gradually add the water, stirring continuously, until smooth. Cook the mixture until thick and add the oil. Whisk the egg whites until stiff. Add the soya mixture, mixing with a fork until well blended but still fluffy.

Heat the oil in a frying pan until really hot. Pour in the egg and soya mixture. Cook gently until the underside is golden brown and the mixture rises a little. Place the pan under a hot grill to cook the top of the omelette. Serve immediately with maple or golden syrup. SERVES 2.

Fillings

Curried Prawn Omelette
Make up a half quantity of the filling for Curried Prawn Ring (page 31) before preparing the omelette. Spoon the hot prawn mixture over the cooked omelette and serve immediately.

Smoked Haddock Omelette
Remove the skin and bones from 225 g/8 oz cooked smoked haddock. Melt 25 g/1 oz margarine in a small saucepan, add the fish and stir in 1 tablespoon chopped parsley. Leave over low heat while you prepare the omelette. Spoon the fish over the omelette, fold over and serve.

Sweet Soufflé Omelette
To make a sweet snack, serve the cooked omelette with maple or golden syrup. Sweet omelettes are also delicious for dessert when a light main course is served.

Desserts

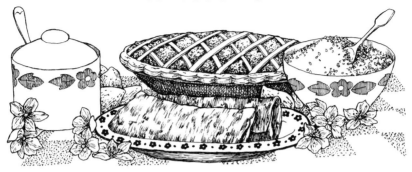

CAROB CUSTARD

25 g/1 oz cornflour
1 tablespoon carob powder
25 g/1 oz sugar

600 ml/1 pint soya milk
50 g/2 oz mixed nuts, chopped

Mix the cornflour, carob powder and sugar in a small bowl. Add a little soya milk to make a thin cream.

Place the rest of the milk in a saucepan and bring to the boil. Pour a little of the boiling milk on to the carob mixture, stirring all the time, then pour this back into the milk in the saucepan.

Return the pan to the heat, stirring all the time, until the mixture thickens. Cook for one minute. Add the nuts and serve in individual bowls.

Carob Mould
Increase the cornflour to 50 g/2 oz and pour the sauce into a mould. Allow to go cold, unmould and serve with canned soya cream.

HAZELNUT MERINGUE CAKE

(Illustrated on page 34)

100 g/4 oz hazelnuts	2 teaspoons cornflour
4 egg whites	pinch of cream of tartar
225 g/8 oz caster sugar	icing sugar

Grease and flour the sides of two 20-cm/8-in sandwich tins and line the bottoms with rounds of non-stick baking paper.

Place the hazelnuts in a moderately hot oven (190c, 375f, gas 5) for 8–10 minutes to brown the nuts. Allow them to cool slightly, then rub off the papery skins. Grind the nuts in a grinder or liquidizer.

Whisk the egg whites until really stiff and dry, then whisk in the sugar, one tablespoonful at a time. Whisk in the cornflour and the cream of tartar. Using a metal spoon, stir in the prepared nuts as lightly as possible.

Divide the mixture between the two tins, level the top, and bake in a moderate oven (180c, 350f, gas 4) for 30–40 minutes until the top is crisp and brown and the inside soft. Allow to cool and turn out on to cooling trays. Allow to go cold before assembling the cake.

Sandwich the two halves of the hazelnut meringue together with Mock Cream (page 111) in the middle and dust the top liberally with sifted icing sugar. SERVES 4–6.

HONEY PANCAKES

100 g/4 oz plain flour	1 tablespoon oil
pinch of salt	honey for spreading
2 egg whites	2 tablespoons sugar
150 ml/$\frac{1}{4}$ pint soya milk	1 teaspoon cinnamon

Place the flour and salt in a bowl. Make a well in the centre and add the two egg whites with a little of the soya milk.

Using a wooden spoon, stir the mixture, bringing in flour from the sides to form a smooth batter. Beat well for 5 minutes, using an electric mixer if preferred.

Stir in the rest of the soya milk and allow the batter to stand for one hour, so that the starch grains soften and the mixture thickens a little. When ready, the batter should be a thick cream which pours easily.

Place the oil in a small frying pan and heat until smoking hot. Pour this oil into the batter mixture and stir well. This makes the batter slightly oily so that there is no need to grease the frying pan after each pancake.

Pour the batter into the pan and roll it around to give a thin layer on the bottom. As the batter goes in it should sizzle and start to cook immediately. If the pan is not hot enough the pancake may stick. When the pancake is set, turn it over and cook the other side. Pile the cooked pancakes on a plate; the oil in the batter will prevent them from sticking.

Spread the pancakes with honey and roll them up. Sprinkle with a mixture of cinnamon and sugar and serve hot. MAKES 6–8.

Note: Maple syrup can be used instead of the honey.

CAROB BAVAROIS

(Illustrated on page 69)

3 tablespoons carob powder
150 ml/¼ pint soya milk
5 teaspoons soya flour
1 tablespoon corn oil
2 tablespoons icing sugar

1½ teaspoons gelatine
2 tablespoons water
100 g/4 oz margarine
2 egg whites

Mix the carob powder with a little of the soya milk to form a thin paste. Place the rest of the milk on the heat. Add the carob mixture and heat through.

Mix together the soya flour and the oil, add this to the soya milk and bring to the boil, stirring all the time. Cook for 2 minutes and stir in the icing sugar.

Place the gelatine and water in a small cup and place the cup in a saucepan of simmering water. Heat until the gelatine is dissolved and clear. Add the dissolved gelatine to the carob mixture and remove from the heat. Add the margarine, a little at a time, and stir until it has all been absorbed.

Whisk the egg whites until stiff and fold them into the carob mixture, so that they are evenly distributed. Pour into individual dishes and allow to set. This is a very rich sweet. SERVES 4–6.

Note: If you like, you can decorate the bavarois with a little chopped or grated Carob bar.

PANTEC PUDDING

1 tablespoon soya flour
2 tablespoons water
2 teaspoons oil
300 ml/½ pint soya milk
2 egg whites, lightly whisked
25 g/1 oz sugar

4 slices bread
margarine
honey
50 g/2 oz almonds, shredded
cinnamon

Mix the soya flour and the water together to form a smooth paste; heat until boiling and cook until thick. Remove from the heat and whisk in the oil until the mixture resembles a pale egg yolk.

To this mixture add the soya milk and the egg whites. Return to the heat and bring to the boil, stirring all the time. Remove from the heat and stir in the sugar.

Remove the crusts from the bread and spread the slices with margarine and honey. Cut each slice into four and arrange them in a greased pie dish. Sprinkle over the almonds and pour over the soya 'custard'. Sprinkle with cinnamon to taste and bake for 30 minutes until set. Serve hot. SERVES 4.

TREACLE TART

175 g/6 oz wholemeal flour
pinch of salt
75 g/3 oz vegetable shortening
2–3 tablespoons water

FILLING
125 g/5 oz golden syrup
100 g/4 oz wholemeal breadcrumbs

Put the flour and salt in a bowl and rub in the fat until the mixture resembles fine breadcrumbs. Stir in the water and make a dough. Because this is such a short pastry, it is best to leave it on one side or in a refrigerator for 30 minutes before rolling out. Roll out the pastry and line a 20-cm/8-in shallow pie plate. Prick the bottom of the pastry.

Warm the golden syrup, add the breadcrumbs, and pour the mixture into the lined pie plate. Roll out the pastry trimmings into strips 6 mm/¼ in wide and use them to make a lattice over the syrup.

Bake the tart in a moderately hot oven (200c, 400f, gas 6) for 25–30 minutes. Serve hot or cold. SERVES 6–8.

MOCK CREAM

15 g/$\frac{1}{2}$ oz cornflour
150 ml/$\frac{1}{4}$ pint soya milk

25 g/1 oz margarine
25 g/1 oz vanilla sugar

Blend the cornflour with a little of the soya milk, and put the rest of the milk on to boil. Pour the boiling soya milk on to the cornflour, stirring all the time. Return the mixture to the pan and cook for 2 minutes until very thick. Cool this mixture.

Cream together the margarine and vanilla sugar until light and fluffy. Gradually beat in the cold cornflour mixture, a little at a time, until the mixture is again light and fluffy.

HONEY DREAMS

(Illustrated on page 51)

4 slices white or brown bread
honey for spreading
2 egg whites

oil for frying
1 tablespoon sugar
1 teaspoon cinnamon

Sandwich the slices of bread together with the honey and press together well. Cut the sandwiches into four triangles and remove the crusts, if desired.

Place the egg whites in a shallow dish and beat until well broken. Heat a little oil in a frying pan. Dip the sandwiches in the beaten egg and immediately fry them in very hot oil until golden brown on both sides. Drain on absorbent kitchen paper.

Mix together the sugar and cinnamon and sprinkle this over the honey dreams. Serve hot. SERVES 2.

Baking

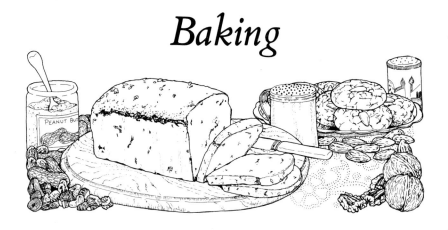

SHORT CRUST PASTRY

175 g/6 oz plain white flour
½ teaspoon salt
75 g/3 oz margarine or vegetable
   shortening

2 tablespoons cold water

Sift the flour into a bowl and add the salt. Rub the fat into the flour until the mixture resembles fine breadcrumbs. Add the water and mix to form a dough. Lightly knead into a ball and use as required.

This is sufficient pastry to line a 20-cm/8-in flan ring or to cover a 1.15-litre/2-pint pie dish.

OAT PASTRY

225 g/8 oz flour
50 g/2 oz rolled oats

100 g/4 oz vegetable shortening
2 tablespoons cold water

Mix together the flour and the oats and rub in the vegetable shortening. Stir in enough cold water to form a dough. Knead lightly and roll out in the usual way. This quantity is sufficient to line a 20-cm/8-in flan tin or to cover a 1.15-litre/2-pint pie dish.

WHOLEMEAL PASTRY

175 g/6 oz wholemeal flour
50 g/2 oz soya flour
pinch of salt

100 g/4 oz margarine or
  vegetable shortening
2 tablespoons water

Mix together the flours, add a pinch of salt and rub in the chosen fat until the mixture resembles fine breadcrumbs. Add just enough water to bind the mixture together.

Wrap the pastry dough in greaseproof paper and leave it in the refrigerator for 30 minutes. This makes the pastry easier to roll out. Roll out the pastry on a floured surface and use as required.

This quantity will cover a 1.15-litre/2-pint pie dish or may be used to line a 20-cm/8-in flan ring.

SAFA CAKE

175 g/6 oz soft margarine
175 g/6 oz caster sugar
4 egg whites
225 g/8 oz semolina

2 teaspoons baking powder
100 g/4 oz ground almonds
1 tablespoon water

Cream the margarine and sugar until light and fluffy. Beat in two of the egg whites, one at a time, beating well to make the mixture as light as possible. Whisk the two remaining egg whites to a foam. Mix together the semolina, baking powder, and ground almonds. Using a metal spoon, fold the dry ingredients into the creamed mixture, then stir in the whisked egg whites. Add a little water to give a dropping consistency.

Line and grease a 23-cm/9-in cake tin. Place the mixture in the tin and spread it evenly. Bake in a moderate oven (180c, 350f, gas 4) for 40 minutes until firm and brown. Allow to cool slightly before removing from the tin, then leave to cool completely on a wire rack. SERVES 8.

MARGO'S BREAD

(Illustrated on page 33)

1 teaspoon sugar
600 ml/1 pint plus 4 tablespoons tepid water
3 teaspoons dried yeast

675 g/1½ lb wholemeal flour
225 g/8 oz strong white flour
1 teaspoon salt

Dissolve the sugar in the 4 tablespoons tepid water, sprinkle over the dried yeast and leave in a warm place for about five minutes or until the yeast has dissolved to give a frothy mixture.

In a large mixing bowl mix the brown and white flours and add the salt. Make a well in the centre of the flour and pour in the yeast mixture. Add the rest of the water. Using a wooden spoon stir the mixture and gradually mix in the flour to make a dough. Remove the dough from the bowl and knead well until it is smooth and elastic. The kneading of the dough strengthens the gluten in the flour, and it is this which gives an evenly-risen, light loaf when baked.

Replace the dough in the bowl, cover with a cloth, and place in a warm place to rise. An airing cupboard is excellent for this. The dough is ready for the next stage when it has doubled in size.

Turn the dough out on to a floured surface. Knead it lightly to distribute the gas bubbles and avoid large holes. Shape the dough into loaves or rolls and place in greased tins. Leave to rise for a further 15 minutes, or until the dough has risen by a third.

Place the loaves in a hot oven (230c, 450f, gas 8) for 15 minutes, then reduce the heat to moderately hot (200c, 400f, gas 6) and cook until the loaves are golden brown and sound hollow when tapped. Large loaves take about one hour to cook and 30 minutes should be allowed for rolls. Remove from the tins and cool on a wire rack.

Note: Once opened, unsealed packets of dried yeast do not have a very long shelf life. If your dried yeast does not froth within about ten minutes it usually means that the yeast is dead.

When available, fresh yeast can be used instead of dried yeast. Allow 25 g/1 oz yeast for the above mixture. Place the yeast in a small basin and add 1 teaspoon sugar. Cream together until runny, then add the 4 tablespoons tepid water and continue as above.

This amount of dough will make two 450 g/1 lb loaves or 24 small bread rolls, or 3 shaped loaves, or any combination of the above.

White Bread
Make as above, using 1 kg/2 lb strong white flour.

PORTADOWN CAKE

(Illustrated on page 88)

175 g/6 oz margarine
175 g/6 oz raw cane sugar
1 tablespoon dandelion coffee *or*
  2 teaspoons instant coffee

1 tablespoon hot water
1 teaspoon baking powder
225 g/8 oz wholemeal flour
2 egg whites

Grease 2 (20-cm/8-in) sandwich tins and flour them lightly.

Cream together the margarine and sugar until light in texture, then beat in the chosen coffee flavouring dissolved in the hot water.

Mix the baking powder with the flour and whisk the egg whites until stiff. Add the egg whites and flour to the creamed mixture. Using a metal spoon, carefully fold the mixture until thoroughly mixed, with an even colour and texture. Try not to over-mix as this will destroy the bulk and lightness in the egg whites.

Divide the mixture between the tins and bake in the centre of a moderately hot oven (190c, 375f, gas 5) for 25–30 minutes. The cake is cooked when the mixture springs back when gently pressed with the finger. Turn out and cool on a wire rack.

When the cakes are cool, sandwich them together with honey or Portadown Cream (see below) and dust the top with icing sugar. SERVES 6–8.

PORTADOWN CREAM

1 tablespoon dandelion coffee *or*
  2 teaspoons instant coffee
1 tablespoon cornflour

150 ml/$\frac{1}{4}$ pint soya milk
50 g/2 oz margarine
1 tablespoon honey

In a small bowl mix together the chosen coffee flavouring and the cornflour. Blend in a little of the soya milk to make a thin cream.

Put the rest of the soya milk on to boil, then pour it into the cornflour mixture. Return this to the saucepan and bring back to the boil, stirring all the time. Remove from the heat and cool.

Cream together the margarine and honey, then gradually beat in the cold cornflour mixture until smooth. Use to sandwich the Portadown Cake, or whenever a cream filling is required.

COFFEE AND WALNUT CAKES

2 egg whites
100 g/4 oz raw cane demerara
   sugar

1 tablespoon instant coffee
25 g/1 oz chopped walnuts

Line a baking sheet with non-stick silicone paper, or greased greaseproof paper.

Place the egg whites in a bowl and add the raw cane sugar. Place the bowl over a pan of boiling water and whisk together until the mixture is really thick and heavy. This mixture is best made with a hand-held electric whisk as it does take 10–15 minutes to make the mixture really thick.

Remove the bowl from the heat and stir in the coffee and the walnuts. Place spoonfuls of the mixture on the baking sheet and bake in a cool oven (150c, 300f, gas 2) for 25–35 minutes. Allow to go cold, then remove from the baking sheet. MAKES 20.

PEANUT BRITTLE

225 g/8 oz granulated sugar

225 g/8 oz peanuts, chopped

Place the sugar in a heavy-based saucepan and place over a high heat. As soon as the sugar starts to melt, reduce the heat then shake the pan so that the sugar melts evenly and turns a light brown. Do not stir the sugar and take care not to over-cook it. It is ready when a small amount dropped into cold water forms a crisp ball.

Grease and line a shallow tin. Sprinkle over the coarsely-chopped peanuts in a single layer. When the sugar is ready, pour it over the peanuts. Allow the brittle to go hard, then break into pieces. Store in an airtight tin.

PEANUT CRUNCHIES

100 g/4 oz margarine
75 g/3 oz brown sugar

50 g/2 oz peanut butter
175 g/6 oz wholemeal flour

Cream the margarine and sugar together until light and fluffy. Beat in the peanut butter and stir in the flour. Knead to make a firm dough, roll out to 5 mm/¼ in thick and cut into fingers.

Bake the fingers on a greased baking sheet in a moderate oven (180c, 350f, gas 4) for 15–20 minutes. Allow to cool before removing from the tray. MAKES 12.

STICKY PARKIN

225 g/8 oz wholemeal flour
450 g/1 lb medium oatmeal
1 teaspoon ground ginger
1 teaspoon cinnamon
1 teaspoon ground mixed spice
pinch of salt

175 g/6 oz margarine
100 g/4 oz raw cane sugar
350 g/12 oz black treacle
½ teaspoon bicarbonate of soda
about 1 tablespoon water or
    soya milk

Line and grease a 23-cm/9-in square baking tin. Mix together the flour, oatmeal, spices and salt. Rub in the margarine until the mixture resembles breadcrumbs. Add the sugar and mix well. Warm the treacle and pour this into the centre of the mixture.

Dissolve the bicarbonate of soda in the water or soya milk and add this to the treacle. Mix well to form a firm dough. Do not add any extra liquid.

Press the dough into the greased tin and bake in a cool oven (150c, 300f, gas 2) for two hours. The parkin is cooked when it feels firm to the touch and shrinks back slightly from the sides of the tin.

Leave to cool in the tin, then cut into squares. MAKES ABOUT 16.

Note: This parkin improves if it is wrapped in greaseproof paper and left for 4–5 days before eating so that the spice flavours mellow and the cake becomes more sticky.

MACAROONS

2 egg whites
175 g/6 oz vanilla sugar
100 g/4 oz ground almonds

25 g/1 oz ground rice
flaked almonds to decorate

Line a baking sheet with silicone (non-stick) paper or rice paper. Remove one teaspoon of the egg white to use as a glaze later and put the rest of the egg whites in a large bowl. Whisk the remaining egg whites until they are stiff and then whisk in the sugar one tablespoon at a time. Use a metal spoon to fold in the ground almonds and ground rice.

Spoon the mixture into twenty small piles on the baking sheet, flatten them out slightly and place a flaked almond on the top of each.

Brush them over with the reserved egg white and bake in a cool oven (150c, 300f, gas 2) for 30 minutes until pale golden. Allow to cool, then remove them from the paper or tear round the rice paper. When they are cold they may be stored in an airtight tin. MAKES 20.

ALEXANDRA BISCUITS

100 g/4 oz raw cane sugar
100 g/4 oz margarine

1 egg white
225 g/8 oz wholemeal flour

Cream the sugar and margarine until very light and fluffy. Add the egg white and beat well. Stir in the flour and mix until a dough is formed.

Divide the mixture into two and roll each piece into a sausage shape 7.5 cm/3 in long. Wrap the dough shapes in greaseproof paper and place in a refrigerator for 30–60 minutes for the dough to become firm.

Slice the rolls into 5-mm/¼-in slices and place them on a greased baking sheet. Prick the biscuits and bake in a moderately hot oven (190c, 375f, gas 5) for 10–15 minutes. Store in an airtight tin when cold. MAKES 24.

Sauces, Salad Dressings
AND BATTERS

MUSHROOM SAUCE

25 g/1 oz margarine
50 g/2 oz mushrooms or
    mushroom stalks, finely
    chopped
25 g/1 oz flour

300 ml/$\frac{1}{2}$ pint vegetable water or
    stock
1 tablespoon soy sauce
salt

Melt the margarine in a small saucepan and add the mushrooms. Cook gently for about 10 minutes but do not let the mushrooms get too brown.

Stir in the flour and cook for a further 2 minutes. Remove from the heat and gradually stir in the vegetable water or stock and the soy sauce. Bring back to the boil to thicken the sauce. Season with salt and serve with fritters or rissoles.

ONION SAUCE

1 tablespoon corn oil
1 medium onion, chopped
1 teaspoon plain flour

150 ml/$\frac{1}{4}$ pint vegetable stock
2–3 teaspoons soy sauce

Heat the oil in a saucepan and fry the onion in it until soft and golden brown. Stir in the flour and cook for two minutes. Remove from the heat and gradually stir in the vegetable stock and the soy sauce. Return the pan to the heat and bring to the boil. Serve with nut cutlets or with any dish which needs a savoury sauce.

BREAD SAUCE

2 cloves
1 small onion
300 ml/$\frac{1}{2}$ pint water or soya milk
blade of mace

100 g/4 oz dry breadcrumbs
15 g/$\frac{1}{2}$ oz margarine
salt

Press the cloves into the onion and place it in a small saucepan with the water or soya milk. Bring to the boil, add the mace and the breadcrumbs. Leave to infuse over very low heat for 30 minutes. Do *not* let the mixture boil.

Remove the onion, cloves and mace; beat in the margarine and salt. Reheat and serve with roast chicken.

PEANUT SAUCE

100 g/4 oz crunchy peanut
    butter
1 tablespoon soy sauce

1 teaspoon honey
1 clove garlic, crushed
$\frac{1}{2}$ teaspoon salt

Mix all the ingredients in a small saucepan and stir in just enough water to make a thick pouring sauce.

Heat, stirring all the time, then serve immediately.

PARSLEY SAUCE

25 g/1 oz margarine
25 g/1 oz flour
300 ml/½ pint court-bouillon
  (see Baked Hake in Oatmeal,
  page 41) *or* soya milk

2 tablespoons chopped fresh
  parsley
salt
nutmeg

Melt the margarine in a small saucepan and add the flour. Cook for 2 minutes without browning the flour and remove the pan from the heat. Gradually stir in the strained court-bouillon, return to the heat and cook, stirring all the time, until the sauce has thickened.

Add the chopped parsley and season with a little salt and nutmeg. Serve with salmon or other fish.

CREAMY SALAD DRESSING

1 tablespoon soya flour
3 tablespoons water

150 ml/¼ pint salad oil
salt

Mix together the soya flour and water to form a paste.

Place the measured oil in a jug and carefully pour it, drop by drop, into the paste. Whisk all the time until the dressing starts to thicken. When the mixture has started to thicken the oil can be added a little faster.

Add a pinch of salt and store in a covered container in the refrigerator. Give the container a good shake before use if the dressing has separated out.

HERB DRESSING

1 tablespoon olive oil
1 teaspoon corn oil
2 teaspoons white wine
salt

2 teaspoons chopped fresh herbs,
  for example parsley, thyme,
  rosemary

Mix together the olive and corn oil and add the wine. Whisk until slightly thick. Season with a pinch of salt and mix in the fresh herbs.

Pour this dressing over the salad vegetables just before serving, and toss lightly.

YEAST BATTER

$\frac{1}{2}$ teaspoon sugar
150 ml/$\frac{1}{4}$ pint tepid water
$\frac{1}{4}$ teaspoon dried yeast
100 g/4 oz plain flour

pinch of salt
1 tablespoon oil
1 small egg white

Dissolve the sugar in the water, sprinkle over the dried yeast and leave in a warm place until frothy.

Sift the flour into a mixing bowl, add the salt, and make a well in the centre. Pour in the yeast mixture and gradually stir to mix the flour and liquid together. Beat the batter until smooth. Cover and leave in a warm place for 30 minutes. Stir in the oil. Whisk the egg white until it is a firm snow and, when the batter is ready for use, fold it in with a metal spoon.

Note: This batter is sufficient to coat four large fillets of fish, 450 g/ 1 lb peeled prawns or 450 g/1 lb vegetable pieces.

BATTER

100 g/4 oz plain flour
salt
25 g/1 oz margarine, melted

150 ml/$\frac{1}{4}$ pint warm water
2 egg whites

Sift the flour and a pinch of salt into a bowl, make a well in the centre, then pour in the melted margarine and the warm water. Mix and beat well until the batter is smooth and bubbles rise to the surface. Leave on one side for at least 20 minutes.

Whisk the egg whites until stiff, then fold them into the batter. Use immediately for coating pieces of fish, vegetables or chicken.

Fry in very hot oil to give a crisp coating.

NUTRIENT CHARTS

Quantities of selected foods which provide an adequate daily intake of vitamins

Vitamin A

broccoli	175 g/6 oz
carrots, new	75 g/3 oz
carrots, old	40 g/1½ oz
chicken	15 g/½ oz
margarine	75 g/3 oz
spinach	75 g/3 oz

Vitamin B$_1$

Brazil nuts	90 g/3½ oz
cod's roe	65 g/2½ oz
flour, wholewheat	200 g/7 oz
peanuts, fresh	100 g/4 oz
peas	300 g/11 oz
wheat germ	50 g/2 oz
yeast	7 g/¼ oz

Vitamin B$_2$ (riboflavin)

almonds	175 g/6 oz
flour, wholewheat	300 g/11 oz
herrings	300 g/11 oz
mackerel	300 g/11 oz
sardines	300 g/11 oz
wheat bran	175 g/6 oz

Vitamin B$_3$ (nicotinic acid)

halibut	175 g/6 oz
mackerel	225 g/8 oz
mushrooms	450 g/1 lb
peanuts, fresh	100 g/4 oz
salmon	200 g/7 oz
sardines	225 g/8 oz

Vitamin B$_6$ (pyridoxine)

avocado	200 g/7 oz
	(about 2 avocadoes)
chicken	200 g/7 oz
wheat germ	25 g/1 oz
yeast	50 g/2 oz

Vitamin B$_{12}$

brisling	25 g/1 oz
egg white	90 g/3½ oz
herrings	25 g/1 oz
pilchards	25 g/1 oz
salmon	90 g/3½ oz
sardines	25 g/1 oz
tuna fish	90 g/3½ oz

Vitamin C (ascorbic acid)

asparagus	100 g/4 oz
avocado	225–350 g/8–12 oz
beans, runner	225–350 g/8–12 oz
broccoli	25 g/1 oz
Brussels sprouts	25 g/1 oz
cabbage, raw	225 g/8 oz
cauliflower	40 g/$\frac{1}{2}$ oz
celery	225–350 g/8–12 oz
green pepper, raw	25 g/1 oz
kale	25 g/1 oz
leeks	225–350 g/8–12 oz
lettuce	225–350 g/8–12 oz
mustard and cress	15 g/$\frac{1}{2}$ oz
parsley	25 g/1 oz
parsnips	225–350 g/8–12 oz
peas	225–350 g/8–12 oz
potatoes, new	100 g/4 oz
potatoes, old	225 g/8 oz
radishes	225–350 g/8–12 oz
spinach	100 g/4 oz
spring onions	225–350 g/8–12 oz
swedes	225–350 g/8–12 oz
watercress	15 g/$\frac{1}{2}$ oz

(**Note**: the above quantities apply to raw vegetables or those boiled in the minimum of water and eaten immediately.)

Vitamin D

cod liver oil	1 teaspoon
cod liver oil and malt	1$\frac{1}{2}$ teaspoons
herrings	100 g/4 oz
margarine	40 g/1$\frac{1}{2}$ oz
salmon	200 g/7 oz
sardines	350 g/12 oz

Quantities of fat and protein obtained from an average portion of selected foods

Fat

bread, wholemeal (100 g/4 oz)	1 g/$\frac{1}{28}$ oz
chicken (100 g/4 oz)	8 g/$\frac{1}{4}$ oz
herrings (100 g/4 oz)	14 g/$\frac{1}{2}$ oz
margarine (25 g/1 oz)	25 g/1 oz
nuts (50 g/2 oz)	28 g/1 oz
soya flour (25 g/1 oz)	6.5 g/$\frac{1}{4}$ oz
vegetable oil (25 g/1 oz)	25 g/1 oz

Protein

bread, wholemeal (100 g/4 oz)	8 g/$\frac{1}{4}$ oz
fish, white (100 g/4 oz)	18 g/$\frac{3}{4}$ oz
nuts (50 g/2 oz)	14 g/$\frac{1}{2}$ oz
potatoes (175 g/6 oz)	2 g/$\frac{1}{14}$ oz
salmon (50 g/2 oz)	11 g/$\frac{1}{4}$–$\frac{1}{2}$ oz
soya milk, diluted (300 ml/$\frac{1}{2}$ pint)	9 g/$\frac{1}{4}$ oz
spun soya (50 g/2 oz)	14 g/$\frac{1}{2}$ oz

(**Note:** The Imperial quantities in the above chart are approximate.)

INDEX